ADVANCE PRAISE FOR *ACHIEVING A GOOD DEATH*

"Chris Palmer has written an important and incredibly useful book designed to give the reader the skills and knowledge to live fully to the end of life and to have a good death. Everyone should read this book and imbibe its wisdom."

—**Steven Petrow, contributing columnist,** *The Washington Post*, **and author of** *Stupid Things I Won't Do When I Get Old*

"As a physician for many years, I wish I had had Chris Palmer's book *Achieving a Good Death* as a resource for my patients and families. He tackles head-on, in a no-nonsense way, the practical issues we all face but generally shy away from dealing with. Each of us deserves a dignified and meaningful end of life, and this book is a sure-fire guide to achieving that noble goal."

—**Kurt Newman, MD, President Emeritus, Children's National Hospital, and author of** *Healing Children: A Surgeon's Stories from the Frontiers of Pediatric Medicine*

"In 1994, Dr. Sherwin Nuland wrote *How We Die*, broke a taboo on books about death, and opened the floodgates. Today, the category is so vast that finding inspiration and answers is daunting. Fortunately, Chris Palmer, an astute and sensitive researcher, has done it all for you, culling, sorting, and presenting the best from many evidence-based sources. Palmer also gives voice to unspoken fears like degradation, pity, and shame, and adds valuable and original suggestions for ethical wills, legacy letters, memoirs, and eulogies from his expertise as a writer and storyteller. Bravo for this eminently helpful and deeply meaningful book."

—**Barbara Coombs Lee, author of** *Finish Strong: Putting Your Priorities First at Life's End*, **and President Emerita/Senior Advisor, Compassion & Choices**

"Chris Palmer's new book presents a compelling exploration into the often avoided yet universally inevitable topic of death and dying. With insightful prose and personal anecdotes, Palmer challenges the sanitized portrayal of death prevalent in media and confronts the taboo surrounding discussions about mortality. As the narrative unfolds, readers are encouraged to embrace the reality of death as a natural part of life, empowering them to approach the end with dignity, agency, and peace. A thought-provoking must-read that invites readers to contemplate the profound meaning of life and the importance of living fully until the very end."

—Mikhail Kogan, MD, Medical Director, GW Center for Integrative Medicine, Associate Professor of Medicine, and Associate Director of Geriatric Fellowship at George Washington University; author of *Integrative Geriatric Medicine*

"Most of us shy away from discussing death and dying, a taboo topic held to be morbid, dark, and depressing. But in his book *Achieving a Good Death*, Chris Palmer sheds light on the elusive 'good death' and provides solid, practical advice for how to take control and have agency in living and dying well. For those of us in the aging field, Palmer's book is a refreshing compliment to his insightful workshops on death and dying. *Achieving a Good Death* belongs in everyone's personal library and should be shared with family and friends."

—Barbara Hughes Sullivan, Executive Director, Village to Village Network

"Achieving a Good Death: A Practical Guide to the End of Life is just EXCELLENT. It addresses all of the areas involved in end-of-life decision-making and educates about the actual dying process and grieving. Comprehensive, direct, and not overly medically phrased, this book is for caregivers, grievers, and those who want a more sacred end-of-life experience."

—Barbara Karnes, RN, hospice pioneer and author of *Gone From My Sight: The Dying Experience*

"Chris Palmer's *Achieving a Good Death* is an exceptional compendium of everything one needs to know to deliberately complete one's life journey with the best chances of avoiding a medicalized death, a ruptured family, and a legacy of grief, second-guessing, and what-ifs. From the medical aspects of dying well to the legal aspects of advance directives, including the social aspects of supporting one's family and caregivers and dealing with the American funeral industry, Palmer covers it all calmly and eloquently. This masterful discussion of all possible end-of-life issues is capped with personalized examples of instructions to physicians about end-of-life wishes and touching examples of ethical wills. Study this carefully; you and your family will undoubtedly benefit from it."

—**Samuel Harrington, MD, author of** *At Peace: Choosing a Good Death After a Long Life*

"Achieving a Good Death by Chris Palmer is a major accomplishment and has the potential to help us all achieve a good death ourselves. I urge everyone to read this book and give it to their friends and family as a gift. Palmer covers every aspect of aging, dying, and death, including death cleaning, ethical wills, memoirs, advance directives, voluntarily stopping eating and drinking, human composting, funeral planning, and more. This book is lucidly written and superbly informed, totally enjoyable, and profoundly wise. I cannot recommend it highly enough."

—**Katrina Spade, founder and CEO of Recompose**

"In this important and inspiring book, Palmer presents a comprehensive and detailed plan for achieving a gentle, humane, and dignified end of life. It is a must-read for anyone who will one day die."

—**Dan Morheim, MD, former Maryland state legislator, emergency-medicine physician, and author of** *Preparing for a Better End*

"Chris Palmer takes the fear, mystery, and anxiety from those facing death and provides practical, informative, and helpful advice to families in their time of need. *Achieving a Good Death* helps honor our loved ones and comfort the bereaved. It should be on the bedstand of every person who will face dying—in other words, everyone. Palmer's outstanding book is a gift to the death care industry and the families we serve."

—**Glenn S. Easton, executive director of the Garden of Remembrance Memorial Park, the first certified Hybrid Green Burial Cemetery in Maryland.**

"This is a must-read for anyone committed to maintaining control of their life to the end. Chris Palmer has covered all the important moments likely to arise in those final days, weeks, and months, making it a comprehensive resource."

—Jessica Nutik Zitter, MD, MPH, Founder of Reel Medicine Media, and author of *Extreme Measures: Finding a Better Path to the End of Life*

"Chris Palmer is a fearless author who expertly leads us into a new and vital vision of death. In *Achieving a Good Death*, as in his previous books, he guides the reader with an expert, thoughtful hand. This topic is universal; the book is essential."

—Lawrence T. Bowles, MD, PhD, former Dean of George Washington University Medical School

"At last, the operator's manual for humans we didn't get at birth—and it's chock full of practical details and insight, written with understanding and humor by a fellow traveler. While many who advise about dying often go silent in the aftermath of the death itself, Chris Palmer plunges right ahead with pinpoint facts and heart-led observations that prepare us in every way for the full possibilities inherent in dying, deathcare, and disposition. I urge you to read this book!"

—Lee Webster, funeral reform advocate, former President of the National Home Funeral Alliance, and co-founder of the National End-of-Life Doula Alliance

"Chris Palmer shares his versatile repertoire of worldly wisdom and practical information about the universal experience of coming to the end of life. Even for those disinclined to do any practical planning, this easy-to-read guide provides key principles that spare our loved ones the agonizing tasks of guessing what kind of personal and medical care we desire if we can no longer articulate our wishes. *Achieving a Good Death* lights our way in the most gentle and reassuring way and should be required reading for all adults!"

—Elizabeth L. Cobbs, MD; Fellow, American Academy of Hospice and Palliative Medicine; Fellow, American Geriatrics Society; Professor, Medicine, Geriatrics, Hospice and Palliative Medicine, George Washington University

"How refreshing to read a prepare-for-the-end guide with the guts to include what so many of us want to know. How do I hasten my death if I'm faced with a future that I find unacceptable? Hats off to Chris Palmer for looking us in the eye and answering."

—Lowrey Brown, Exit Guide Program Director for Final Exit Network

"Just when you think it's safe to bypass the 'Death and Dying' section at your local bookstore or library . . . Kudos to Chris Palmer, who has penned a remarkable compendium of what all of us need to know in order to die well. Read this book, then buy an extra copy for your family and friends."

—Sara Williams, President, Funeral Consumers Alliance

"Chris Palmer somehow provides a comforting approach to a traditionally unapproachable topic. He soothes daunting fears about death and aging and turns them into a source of motivation to strive for a full, intentional, and present life. I'm a big fan of Chris Palmer's work across his breadth of topics and am especially grateful for *Achieving a Good Death*. This book is so important and near and dear to my heart. It gives me the bravery to dig deep enough and go for what I truly want and the guidance for considering the wishes of my loved ones—now through the end of life."

—Cyn Meyer, author of *From Aimless to Amazing: The Rewire Retirement Method* and founder of Second Wind Movement

"In a comprehensive but highly readable format, Chris Palmer has addressed all the concerns, issues, and questions that friends, colleagues, and patients typically raise regarding the end of life—well done."

—Michael J. Strauss, MD, MPH, President, Marylanders for End-of-Life Options

"Chris Palmer thoughtfully captures the depth and breadth of this hard and holy conversation we all fear to have, and yet without it, a good death is surely denied. Everyone who will die should read this book and take its profound message to heart. You only die once. This manual will better ensure we don't mess it up. Give to your parents, your adult children, your clinicians, and your clergy. Give it to those you love and who love you."

—Dixcy Bosley, RN, MSN, FNP, clinical nurse care manager, hospice nurse, and end-of-life activist

"Chris Palmer's new book, *Achieving a Good Death,* deserves a place on your bookshelf as a classic next to Elisabeth Kübler-Ross's *On Death and Dying.* He shows us that 'death encourages us to live our best life' and offers practical advice on how to do so. Palmer provides invaluable guidance about advance directives, the 'hard conversation' about end-of-life care, hospice, palliative care, 'green burials' and other eco-friendly body disposition choices, and many other topics. Everyone should read this profoundly insightful book."

—Dick Jung, creator and author of the multimedia biography, *Michael Kirst: An Uncommon Academic*

"Chris Palmer's comprehensive, easy-to-read guide covers everything you need to know before you go. We are all going to die, so use it to help your loved ones today!"

—Gail Rubin, CT, author of A Good Goodbye: Funeral Planning for Those Who Don't Plan to *Die*

"Chris Palmer has written an invaluable guide to the overwhelming decisions that most of us run from until we find ourselves facing the inevitable. He sets out crystal-clear options for everything from household decluttering and end-of-life care to a surprisingly broad array of burial choices. His courageous, unflinching guidance brings the seemingly unfathomable within our grasp."

—Philip Warburg, former president of the Conservation Law Foundation and author of *Harvest the Wind* and *Harness the Sun*

"Those of us who desire a peaceful, dignified, and compassionate end-of-life experience must read Chris Palmer's new book, *Achieving a Good Death.* Having a sensitive guide at the end of life is extremely helpful, and Chris Palmer is the perfect guide. This book provides the tools to navigate the challenging final chapter of life. Please read it and pass it on!"

—David Schrier, MD, Chief Medical Office, Montgomery Hospice and Prince George's Hospice

"Chris Palmer, a popular guest on the Positive Aging Discussion Series, offers readers a comprehensive guide in his book, *Achieving a Good Death*. This book is a valuable resource for those seeking a peaceful and dignified end-of-life experience. Palmer's insights and practical advice provide comfort and clarity, making it an essential read for anyone navigating the complexities of aging and end-of-life planning."

—Steve Gurney, Founder and Director of the Positive Aging Community

"Chris Palmer's *Achieving a Good Death* takes an often daunting topic and makes it wonderfully approachable. Through a deeply personal and well-researched approach, he demystifies the steps necessary to exit the world without fear of loose ends. Palmer does a masterful job of providing a comprehensive yet easily digestible overview of what constitutes a good death. As an end-of-life physician, I highly recommend this book to help guide patients facing the great beyond."

—Donald Moore, MD, End-of-Life Physician and founder of Eumoria Health.

"This book on end-of-life concerns, questions, decisions, and opportunities is a gem! It is a comprehensive but easy read, well organized, and indeed practical. Chris Palmer is a clear, well-reasoned voice in our ongoing societal conversations about dying with dignity, autonomy, and comfort. He stresses the key importance of conversations and advance planning, moves through the various options for a good death, and then covers the new variety of options for burial. It is probably the best, most straightforward book I've read on this topic!"

—The Rev. Susan Flanders, Episcopal Priest and the author of *If I Ever Lose My Mind: Aid in Dying With Advanced Dementia*

"An *essential* new book about an age-old topic. *Achieving a Good Death* won't save your life, but it just might save you from one of the many ways in which it is possible to die badly (all documented in detail in the book).

If you're currently in your senior years, I have one thing to say: 'You owe it to yourself to read this book!'"

—Dr. Mardy Grothe, author of *Oxymoronica, I Never Metaphor I Didn't Like*, and other books.

"As a physician and now a natural cemeterian, dealing with death has been a difficult topic to discuss. In Chris Palmer's book, *Achieving A Good Death*, he is able to carefully walk us through fears we may face and educate us along the way to make the process meaningful and peaceful."

—Howard K. Berg, MD, owner of the Serenity Ridge Natural Burial Cemetery

"Achieving a Good Death is an extraordinary guide for completing a purposeful, enjoyable, fulfilling, and meaningful life until the very last of our days. It also helps us to create a legacy that will have a lasting impact on those we love. This masterpiece of a book is about LIFE and LOVE. Palmer summarizes everything we must do to relish life until the last minute. He shares many first-hand examples of how to accomplish it. Our favorite tip: Toast letters. What a gift this book is! Don't wait—it's always too late but never too early to start your own journey!"

—Nacho Moreno and Farah Baxter, founders of www.soalma.com— the legacy planning and sharing platform

"At a time when we feel increasingly unable to deal with death, there are few opportunities to contemplate our inescapable expiration date. In elegant prose and with clarity and compassion, Chris Palmer's book *Achieving a Good Death* offers just such an opportunity. Making a graceful departure is a choice we all have. But as Palmer argues, getting it right depends on how we approach the hard questions. In this book, he eloquently shows us how."

—Sarah Murray, author of *Making an Exit: From the Magnificent to the Macabre—How We Dignify the Dead*

"The world needs more Chris Palmers, helping us turn our fleeting attention to the wonder of life and its ends. Fortunately for us, he's written this book."

—BJ Miller, MD, Co-Founder of Mettle Health and Author of *A Beginner's Guide to the End*

"Achieving a Good Death: A Practical Guide to the End of Life is a comprehensive exploration of death and dying in America, covering both the philosophical and the practical. Author Chris Palmer serves as a humane and knowledgeable guide to our final days. He eloquently shares his personal journey making end-of-life plans and coming to terms with mortality, inspiring readers to confidently navigate the many endings in their own lives. His book is an engaging read cover to cover and a handy reference I will revisit again and again."

—Sarah Weinstein, Executive Director, Hemlock Society of San Diego

ACHIEVING A GOOD DEATH

ACHIEVING A GOOD DEATH

A Practical Guide to the End of Life

CHRIS PALMER

ROWMAN & LITTLEFIELD
Lanham • Boulder • New York • London

Published by Rowman & Littlefield
An imprint of The Rowman & Littlefield Publishing Group, Inc.
4501 Forbes Boulevard, Suite 200, Lanham, Maryland 20706
www.rowman.com

86-90 Paul Street, London EC2A 4NE

British Library Cataloguing in Publication Information Available

Library of Congress Cataloging-in-Publication Data
Names: Palmer, Chris, author.
  Title: Achieving a good death: a practical guide to the end of life / Chris Palmer.
  Description: Lanham : Rowman & Littlefield, [2024] | Includes index.
  Identifiers: LCCN 2024006725 (print) | LCCN 2024006726 (ebook) | ISBN
      9781475850512 (cloth) | ISBN 9781475850529 (ebook)
  Subjects: LCSH: Death--Psychological aspects. | Death--Social aspects. |
      Death. | Terminal care.
  Classification: LCC BF789.D4 P34 2024 (print) | LCC BF789.D4 (ebook) |
      DDC 155.9/37--dc23/eng/20240527
  LC record available at https://lccn.loc.gov/2024006725
  LC ebook record available at https://lccn.loc.gov/2024006726

♾️™ The paper used in this publication meets the minimum requirements of American National Standard for Information Sciences—Permanence of Paper for Printed Library Materials, ANSI/ NISO Z39.48-1992.

For my beloved wife of nearly fifty years, Gail Shearer

Contents

CONTENTS

Other Books by Chris Palmer

Shooting in the Wild: An Insider's Account of Making Movies in the Animal Kingdom (Sierra Club Books, 2010)

Confessions of a Wildlife Filmmaker: The Challenges of Staying Honest in an Industry Where Ratings Are King (Bluefield Publishing, 2015)

Now What, Grad? Your Path to Success after College (Rowman & Littlefield, 2015)

Raise Your Kids to Succeed: What Every Parent Should Know (Rowman & Littlefield, 2017)

Now What, Grad? Your Path to Success after College, 2nd Edition (Rowman & Littlefield, 2018)

Love, Dad: Letters from a Father to His Daughters (Bethesda Communications Group, 2018)

College Teaching at Its Best: Inspiring Students to Be Enthusiastic, Lifelong Learners (Rowman & Littlefield, 2019)

Open Heart: When Open-Heart Surgery Becomes Your Best Option (Bethesda Communications Group, 2021)

Finding Meaning and Success: Living a Fulfilled and Productive Life (Rowman & Littlefield, 2021)

PREFACE

Whenever I told people I was writing a book on death and dying, their typical reaction was perplexity. Why would anyone spend time on such a gloomy and morbid topic? But there is an art to dying well that can be taught and learned. While death is inevitable, dying badly is not. This book is about achieving a good death.

In writing this practical guide to the end of life, I hope to reduce the fear that often cloaks discussions about death and dying.[1] I have loosely organized the book on the continuum from life to death:

The *Preface* (what you are reading now) describes how I have organized the book.

The *Introduction* describes the book's purpose and my journey into death and dying.

Chapter 1 defines a good death and explains why it's elusive.

Chapter 2 focuses on how to live well so as to die well.

Chapter 3 describes how to declutter so we don't burden our loved ones with a big mess when we die.

Chapter 4 discusses the importance of talking with our loved ones and doctors about our wishes and aspirations at the end of life so they know what matters to us and how we want to be treated.

Chapter 5 focuses on our legacy. We live on after we die in the legacy we leave behind. Writing a legacy letter (an ethical will) and a memoir lets our loved ones know what is deep in our hearts.

Chapter 6 examines caregivers, an underappreciated group of people, usually unpaid women, who number in the millions.

Chapter 7 explores the benefits of palliative care, hospice, and end-of-life doulas and the necessary vigilance to get the most out of these essential services.

Chapter 8 describes various end-of-life options, including medical aid in dying (MAID) and voluntarily stopping eating and drinking (VSED).

Chapter 9 explores what it is like to die and how to help people as they die.

Chapter 10 focuses on the disposition of the body of a loved one (or your own body) after death.

Chapter 11 discusses ways to commemorate and celebrate a person's life.

Chapter 12 explores grief, what it is, how to deal with it, and why it is often unbearably painful.

The *Epilogue* is about reimagining death and dying and exploring ways to reinvent the end of life so we think about it constructively rather than letting it fill us with anxiety.

Appendix I provides examples of letters describing a desired end of life.

Appendix II provides examples of legacy letters and ethical wills.

Appendix III provides an example of a eulogy.

Appendix IV provides an example of a burial and memorial service.

I hope this book will give you the knowledge and skills to achieve a peaceful and gentle death.

Introduction

In the television drama *Downton Abbey*, Violet Crawley, Dowager Countess of Grantham, played by Maggie Smith, was a significant source of comedic barbs and repartees. The matriarch was always prepared to let loose with a withering one-liner. In the spin-off Hollywood film *Downton Abbey: A New Era* (2022), we see the dowager on her deathbed, an emotional high point of the film. As she dies peacefully, she delivers one final funny zinger. She gently chides Denker, her lady's maid, "Stop crying, Denker. I can't hear myself die."

While effective dramatically, the scene in the film gives viewers a misleading impression of what death is typically like in reality. Deaths like the dowager's, marked by peace, no pain, and full cognitive alertness right up to the last breath, are rare. Dr. BJ Miller and Shoshana Berger write, "Staying conscious right up to the time of death usually isn't possible, no matter how determined you are." They add, "Common occurrences, such as kidney and liver failure, delirium, or infection, will alter your consciousness."[1]

Television and Movies Portray Dying Unrealistically

Television and movies generally misrepresent death, especially of older people, and portray dying in an absurd fairy-tale way, as we see in the death of the dowager. While it would have been inappropriate to show this in the Downton Abbey film, a more realistic portrayal of Violet's death might have included the symptoms common to the end of life: agitation, delirium, confusion, cognitive decline, nausea, death rattles, pain, irregular and labored breathing, loss of urine and stool control, unconsciousness, change in skin color, bedsores, and, finally, the mouth hanging open when death arrives. In reality, as opposed to in British fictional historical dramas, indignities abound for a dying person.

The death scene in *Downton Abbey* is the tip of a sanitizing iceberg. From movies and television, we have become accustomed to seeing death as fast, simple, and pain-free. This is quite misleading. Death is frequently slow, disturbing, smelly, disagreeable, and noisy. Violet's death also hides a contradiction. In real life, dying is an intense, emotional experience as we face physical extinction and the loss of consciousness. But it's also an experience marked by tedium, monotony, a shrinking world, and dull routines as our vitality ebbs away.

DEATH IS A TABOO TOPIC

We watch staged death for entertainment but recoil from actual death. In her book *Making an Exit*, author Sarah Murray points out that our relationship with death is schizophrenic. She writes, "On the one hand, we hide mortality behind a curtain of medical procedures, materialism, and euphemisms. On the other hand, we parade it across cinema and TV screens in its goriest incarnations."[2]

In 2017, I created a shared-interest group in our village to discuss aging, death, and dying and gave it a straightforward name: "The Aging, Death, and Dying Shared Interest Group." But some members told me, "People don't want to see the words death and dying." They were worried that those words would stress and repel potential new members of the village. So, I reluctantly changed the name to the "Aging Well" group.[3] I write "reluctantly" because one of my goals with the group was to get us to face the fact that we will all die. The mortality rate never dips below 100 percent. Removing those two words seemed to undermine the mission.

It's rational to fear death. Death is mysterious, scary, and dark. We fear what might happen to our bodies, we fear no longer being able to care for those we love, and we worry about our projects not getting finished. Moreover, our death will likely lead to grief and suffering for those who love us, and dying might be painful. And we will no longer be able to undertake adventures, new relationships, or new experiences.

Death and dying are taboo topics, so we don't discuss them and often arrive at the end of our lives unprepared and vulnerable to not being treated the way we want. Americans tend to view death and dying with much trepidation and to see it as defeat and failure. The British philosopher of history Arnold Toynbee once said, only half-jokingly, that death was "un-American."[4]

We deny death and turn our heads away from the suffering and loneliness that accompany dying. Death has become an unfamiliar phenomenon and a more remote experience for people. As a result, it has become inappropriate in polite society to talk about dying and death, except in the most superficial way. We gently stifle and suppress conversations about the end of life. Talking about death and dying is looked down upon as unseemly and tasteless. People who discuss the topic are viewed as morbid and unwelcome. Talk of death tends to kill conversation rather than enliven it.

In his book, *The Best Care Possible*, Dr. Ira Byock, a prominent palliative care doctor and author, writes, "The subject of how we die is depressing. . . . Our cultural tendency is to avoid serious conversations about the end of life. Pain, pus, puking, being at the mercy of doctors, the astronomical expenses, the utter disruption of life. Who wants to think about any of that?"[5] It's natural to want to avoid serious conversations about the end of life.

DEATH USED TO BE A COMMUNITY EVENT

Most people died at home in the nineteenth and early twentieth centuries, so almost everyone was familiar with death. As late as 1910, more than 85 percent of Americans died at home.[6] It would be a common experience for people to be aware of a situation in their neighborhood where a person was dying, perhaps in pain, in an upstairs bedroom. Death was a family and community event. Our forebears had rituals and customs to help guide them. Dying people were surrounded by loved ones and comforted by candles and prayers. Bedside vigils were common. Once the person died, the body would be washed and dressed. Church bells would toll, and the neighbors and community would gather around the family.

In contrast, modern generations are unfamiliar with death and have little practice in dealing with it. We struggle to make it a sacred rite of passage. Many people die in a hospital or nursing home where dead bodies are quickly put in body bags and taken away on a gurney as if dying were a social blunder that shouldn't happen in polite society.

How Dying and Death Have Changed

Before the 1950s, deaths were predominantly from accidents or acute diseases that typically killed people relatively quickly. Our final illnesses didn't last long. Infections like pneumonia caused most deaths. There was only a small involvement from health-care providers and technology.

Today, 80 to 90 percent of deaths are from chronic diseases, such as heart disease, stroke, cancer, diabetes, or dementia, and are protracted, with doctors and medical technology highly involved. Dying is mainly done by older people unless it's by accident, drug overdose, suicide, or violence. Those causes of death tend to happen to younger people. Hospitals and medical progress have advanced so much that doctors can defer death, prolong life, and cure disease using medical marvels, such as organ transplants, chemotherapy, and radiation.

Most of Us Will Die Slowly and Uncomfortably

Most of us in the modern world will die slowly in old age of chronic, incurable illnesses, and we don't know how to handle and deal with these painfully slow deaths, sometimes lasting years. Unlike one hundred years ago, when death was usually a sudden catastrophe, today, it's a drawn-out, slow, lingering, and torturous affair. Many deaths are hidden and invisible. As people die, they're often isolated and alone, shut away in intensive-care units (ICUs) or nursing homes to protect the rest of us from death's sights, sounds, and smells.

Medicine has made life longer while, at the same time, making dying more prolonged and often harrowing. We have delayed death but also made arriving at death more arduous. Dying slowly can often be worse than death. For the most part, dying is a lengthy medical procedure rather than a sacred and hallowed life event.

Euphemisms Are Part of the Problem

People (including doctors) often resort to euphemisms and circumlocutions because to say someone "died" or is "dead" is to be too blunt, too candid, and too uninhibited. In addition, we fear death and dying, so we use euphemisms to avoid having to say the D word and to keep death and dying at an emotionally comfortable distance.

We say he "passed," or "passed away," or "she is no longer with us," or the patient "expired." Or, more colloquially, we say a patient or loved one finally "gave up the ghost," "was lost," or "shuffled off their mortal coil." The flippant might say a person "kicked the bucket," "bought the farm," or "croaked." Religious people might say the deceased has "gone to meet his maker" or "crossed over" or "is resting in peace." Funeral homes like to use the word "transitioned." Doctors and bureaucratic health-care providers might say a dead patient experienced a "negative patient-care outcome" or "multiple organ systems failure."

All these euphemistic ways of saying "a person died" reveal our fear of death and our desire to deny it. We call death by softer names because we fear that saying the word "death" is to encourage or even invite it. We fear not only death but also the pain and deterioration that precedes it. We don't want to suffer while dying. Isaac Asimov said, "Life is pleasant. Death is peaceful. It's the transition that's troublesome."

Euphemisms enable us to continue being timid in discussing end-of-life issues. Instead, we must reduce the taboo of discussing death and dying. We can do better than react with prudishness, evasion, and withdrawal to the one challenge we all will face. We need to defang death and unfetter our minds from fear by talking about death and dying less self-consciously. We must recognize death as a normal and natural event.

Death Encourages Us to Live Our Best Life

No one escapes death. Many of us don't want to think about it and tend to turn away in discomfort from the topic if it comes up in conversation. But, for a few, and I count myself among them, death is frequently on their minds for positive and constructive reasons. Remembering we will die (memento mori) helps us to live more fully, to clarify what matters to us, and to extract every ounce of meaning and joy from our short time on earth.

Remembering that we will die helps us to not take tomorrow for granted and to be grateful for each day as it miraculously unfolds. The inevitability of death reminds us not to squander our lives on meaningless distractions. The fact that life is transitory softens our hearts and allows us to feel awe and wonder. This is why we prize a glorious setting sun or a rose at its zenith of beauty.

By facing death, we learn about life and the preciousness of being alive. The death-care pioneer Elisabeth Kübler-Ross once said, "It is the denial of death that is partly responsible for people living empty, purposeless lives; for when you live as if you will live forever, it becomes too easy to postpone the things you know you must do."[7]

Like most people, I don't want to die. I love life intensely. My fear of death led me to avoid thinking about it for years. I pretended it was never going to happen. But as I got into my sixties and seventies (I'm now seventy-six), my fear of death led me in a new and unusual direction: I wanted to confront it, to understand it, to dig deeply into it to find its meaning and purpose, and to be less intimidated by it. This book is one of the results of that search. Knowing I will not live forever helps me cherish what is important: my relationships, nurturing my family and friends, and finding meaning and purpose in life.

THE DEATH OF FAMILY MEMBERS

One experience that sparked my interest in death and dying was watching my parents and three brothers die. All five deaths involved significant and unnecessary pain and suffering. My mother languished in a nursing home for four years before dying. A woman of great vitality, warmth, and humor, she suffered in this degraded condition, slowly deteriorating, having to wear a diaper, be cleaned by aides, and watch television all day.

My father, whom I admired and loved, died of prostate cancer. Our goodbye was nothing like the intimate moment I had wished for. In the hospital room, I asked him how he was feeling. The next day, I clumsily asked the same question. "I told you yesterday," he snapped irritably.[8]

My three brothers died unexpectedly (and in intense pain) from heart disease at relatively young ages (forty-six, seventy-two, and seventy-five). Their deaths and those of my parents lacked community and family involvement. We handed everything off to professionals, and the family was relegated to a relatively passive role. We also had scant discussion of what they wanted at the end of their lives. We didn't spend time saying thank you and whispering tender goodbyes. And we didn't take time to reflect on the sacredness of their deaths.

There was so much I didn't know about the end of the lives of my parents and brothers. Did they get sufficient pain control? Did they feel abandoned in any way or lonely? Did they have conflicts or frustrations with others (including me) that I should have helped resolve? Did they have regrets over not having lived the lives they wanted? Did they find any purpose in their dying? Did they consider how they wanted to dispose of their bodies? Did they endure unnecessary suffering because of futile and excessive medical interventions? Did they thank the people they wanted to thank for all the love and help they had been given in their lives?

What I took away from observing the deaths of my family members is that we need a better and more humane approach to helping people achieve good deaths, especially older people with chronic diseases. Dying is not the worst thing that can happen to us. The worst thing is when dying robs us of what it means to be human, such as being able to cherish our friends and loved ones.

Our dying is important because it's the last memory we leave with our loved ones. Unfortunately, my last memories of my parents and brothers were not good. I'm determined to do better at the end of my life. As Dr. Ira Byock pointed out in his book *The Best Care Possible*, "There are worse things than having someone you love die . . . there is having the person you love die badly, suffering as they die. Worse still is realizing later that much of their suffering was unnecessary."[9]

Fascination with Death Is Not Morbid
If my fascination with death and dying strikes you as dour and morbid—or even intentionally irrational or perverse—then remember that

an interest in death means, in part, doing everything we can to avoid protracted suffering and deterioration as we approach the end of our lives. That is the epitome of rationality and common sense.

Rather than being morbid or macabre, curiosity about death and dying is fundamentally about making the most of life as we approach death—and living fully right up to the end. How can we achieve a good life and the best possible end of life? Searching for an answer is not morbid but life-affirming and involves embracing life with intentionality and energy.

I agree with language and quotation expert Dr. Mardy Grothe, who, when reflecting on his death, wrote, "Do I find the thought of dying depressing? Hell no! On the contrary, knowing that my Estimated Time of Departure is getting closer just deepens my resolve to pursue the many projects that have given such a great deal of meaning to my life."[10]

SLOW VERSUS FAST DEATH

Author and nurse Barbara Karnes says there are only two ways to die: suddenly (unanticipated and unattended) or slowly (anticipated and attended). Of the 2.5 million people who die in the United States every year, most of us (80 to 90 percent) will die slowly, with time to get to know what will bring our lives to an end.[11] Only 10 to 20 percent of us will die fast without any warning (for example, in a car accident).

Slow death allows us to make some choices, such as where to die, how much treatment to have, and how to spend the limited time we have left. In addition, slow death gives us time to shape our legacy and declutter our possessions. We can be clear about our goals of care and how we want the end of our lives to unfold. A slow death lets us focus on what matters as we enter the last phase of our lives.

THE COVID-19 PANDEMIC AND DEATH

I began working on this book many years before the pandemic started in March 2020. COVID-19 made a mockery of a good death. Too many people, especially older people, died badly. They died on a ventilator, unable to speak, cared for by nurses hidden by multiple masks and gowns, and able to communicate with loved ones only through screens. My mother-in-law died this way in 2020 from COVID-19. It was awful.[12]

According to the Lancet Commission on the Value of Death, which released its first report in January 2022, the pandemic did not change our attitudes toward death and dying. It did not bring a greater acceptance of death. On the contrary, the Commission saw evidence of the opposite. Governments tried to reduce the number of deaths (not the amount of suffering); emphasis was placed on ventilators and intensive care (and little on palliative care[13]); bereavement was overlooked; anxiety about death and dying was increased; and death and dying came to belong still more to health care, with families and loved ones excluded.[14]

Peaceful and Dignified Death

People typically want a peaceful and dignified death. This book will help readers navigate the end of life, keep their priorities straight as illness and aging advance, and avoid landing unintentionally on what palliative care doctor Jessica Zitter calls "a conveyor belt" of unnecessary surgeries or other treatments that lead to miserable intubated deaths in the ICU.[15]

Many people do not want to become demented, incontinent, and dependent on others for daily toileting and other activities. They fear a long and painful decline. They want to live joyfully and vibrantly and then have a swift, painless, and gentle death.

I believe people should have choices at the end of life. This book describes how to achieve a quality end-of-life experience marked by grace, agency, and peace, and on terms that the dying patient wants. We must reform and redesign end-of-life care and pursue patient-directed care.

The Purpose of This Book

My goal in this book is to show that we have multiple options at the end of life and can design, control, and direct our end-of-life journey. Unfortunately, too many doctors think that longevity is all that patients care about, regardless of the pain and suffering. However, a 2017 poll found that 75 percent of people care more about the quality of their lives than the length. Rather than longevity, most people care about dying at home, being at peace spiritually, and being free of pain.[16] This book aims to help people die well when the time comes and shows how to have a life as fulfilling and meaningful as possible right up to the end.

DISCLAIMER

This book does not aim to provide specific medical or legal advice. Where specific medical advice is necessary or appropriate, please consult with an experienced and competent doctor. This book is not a substitute for consulting with your doctor, who is knowledgeable about your specific symptoms, situation, medical condition, and circumstances. Similarly, legal issues and decisions should be discussed with your lawyer.

TWO APOLOGIES

First, an apology to those who don't have families and so may feel left out of the book's narrative with its emphasis on families, children, and grandchildren. And a second apology to those who believe in a spiritual life beyond bodily death and may feel the book does not sufficiently acknowledge such beliefs. My aim is to inform, help, and respect all readers.

CHAPTER 1

What Is a Good Death?

"The last act is bloody, however delightful the rest of the play may be," Blaise Pascal wrote in his *Pensées* (1670). And while it's true that some people die badly—lonely, isolated, in pain, and even in despair—it doesn't have to be that way.

These pages will argue that a last act can be marked by serenity, acceptance, love, comfort, a sense of completeness, and a final departure in which one is surrounded by loving friends and family members.

Good Death in the Civil War Era

In 1861, the United States engaged in a civil war that killed 750,000 Americans in an unprecedented carnage. The deaths were horrendous, especially because the slaughter on the battlefields invariably led to gross violations of the prevailing beliefs about what made a good death.

The concept of the good death was widely accepted in Civil War–era America. Dying was an art with its own traditions and rules. People had assumptions and strong feelings about the proper way to die, and those assumptions clashed badly with the reality of battlefield butchery.

Historian Drew Gilpin Faust vividly explored how death transformed society and culture in her book, *This Republic of Suffering: Death and the American Civil War*. For the first time, civilians confronted the reality of death and maiming from war because of the new technology of photography.

Soldiers and their families found the most distressing aspect of death in the Civil War was that so many combatants were dying far from home.

This caused intense pain because the family was a vital component of a good death, as understood by Americans in the Civil War era. A person should end life among family gathered around the deathbed. Family members wanted to witness a death "in order to assess the state of the dying person's soul, for these critical last moments of life would epitomize his or her spiritual condition."[1]

We can see that some elements of a good death from more than 150 years ago are still in play today. For example, surveys show that most people want to die at home surrounded by their loved ones.[2]

A GOOD DEATH TODAY

A good death in the twenty-first century is a death the dying person wants. It is deeply personal and subjective and aligned with the desires and values of the dying individual. Someone of unwavering Catholic faith might find redemption through enduring suffering. Another might opt for every possible medical intervention. Someone else might define a good death as having the autonomy to decide when to transition to hospice care. Each individual will have a distinct vision of what constitutes a good death.[3]

For many, a good death is gentle, peaceful, free of pain and suffering, and full of grace and dignity. The dying person is surrounded by loved ones, has a chance to say goodbye and thank them, and hears from those present how much the dying person's life meant to them. The room is full of loving exchanges, expressions of tenderness and gratitude, perhaps joyful reconciliations, and shared memories of a well-lived life.

A good death is characterized by doctors telling the patient honestly that death is near so the patient can say goodbye. Talking openly about death's inevitability does not make it more likely to happen. Instead, it allows patients to complete their lives with grace, gratitude, and expressions of love and appreciation and focus on what matters to them.

A good death requires other people to be present. Until the very end, a dying patient needs support from others, including loved ones, friends, and hospice and palliative care providers. Dying is a human and social affair, not simply a medical event. A good death requires help and input from many people.

A good death means being prepared to die, having few regrets, and having one's affairs in order. It means to have one's advance directive followed and to be able to die when one wants to. Above all, a good death means the dying patient controls what is happening to him.

Defining a good death is challenging because it is highly individual and subjective and may change over time. In 2006, nurse and researcher Karen Kehl carefully analyzed the concept of a good death and concluded that five important qualities need to be present:

1. Control and agency over one's treatment, including the ability to decline medical interventions if desired;

2. Comfort and having no pain;

3. Closure and the opportunity to reconcile with family and friends and to make one's memory a blessing;

4. Affirmation and being valued and appreciated for one's life and legacy;

5. Trust that dying and death are appropriate with advanced age and disease and that one trusts one's caregivers and medical providers.[4]

IS "GOOD DEATH" AN OXYMORON?

Is a "good death" an oxymoron, a ludicrous and unacceptable contradiction? After all, a "good" death suggests a "good" time leading up to death, but how can dying ever be good when it's the end of life? How can the greatest loss we experience ever be described as "good"? Deaths are mostly extremely sad as someone much loved is gone forever.

The answer is that there is a significant difference between dying peacefully in your bed at home and dying yoked to tubes and machines in an ICU, receiving futile care that only prolongs the dying process for perhaps a few days while providing a horrendous quality of life.

While, in a real sense, no death is ever "good," planning and preparation can make death less awful and painful.

TWO DIFFERENT DEATHS

Why is it that some people die badly and some people die well? Of course, age, disease, and treatment are all factors, but a significant role is played by the life the person has lived. Author and activist Barbara Coombs Lee's book *Finish Strong: Putting Your Priorities First at Life's End* describes the death of two older men.

Otto was in constant pain, liked to smoke, and was dying of advanced emphysema. He had no family or friends. He did not acknowledge his death in any way. He made no effort to put his affairs in order or plan for his death. He had a shockingly impoverished life and died alone.

In contrast, Nate was dying of heart disease, and his doctor had the gumption to let him die peacefully without any aggressive medical interventions. Nate had been a popular history teacher at his local high school and was now in his midseventies. The doctors and nurses removed all the wires and tubes from Nate, took him off all the whirring machines, bathed him, made him comfortable, and told his family stationed outside his room to come in and bid him goodbye.

One by one, they came in for a final, intimate conversation, telling him how much they loved him, what he meant to them, and how they would tell his story to their children and grandchildren. His death, when it came, was "just as gentle as a leaf falling from a tree."[5]

Coombs Lee was stunned by the radically different deaths of Otto and Nate and concluded that death itself is not the biggest problem people fear. A far bigger fear is the terror of never having lived, of wasted lives and squandered opportunities to make giving, generosity, and gratitude the bedrock of one's life.[6]

Life and death are intertwined. Living impacts dying. Awareness of death reminds us that we are only here temporarily. Life is fragile; that is the nature of the human condition. Death can come at any time.

When we live and love fully (i.e., engage in activities that are meaningful to us and have relationships with people we care about and who care about us), then we are more likely to experience a good death. Coombs Lee writes, "Girded with the fullness of a life well-lived, people could die unafraid, as Nate did."[7]

What Does a "Bad" or "Hard" Death Look Like?

The answer to that question depends on the dying patient's values, preferences, and priorities. For some, having their backsides wiped by a nursing aide is no big deal, while it is an intolerable indignity for others. For some, as long as they can watch television, then life is worth living, while, for others, being in an ICU away from home, unable to talk with family and friends due to intubation, and unable to pursue meaningful projects, makes life a nightmare.

A bad death might mean the dying person experiences excruciating pain that is not treated adequately. Inadequately treated pain can come in many forms, including delirium, difficulty breathing, anxiety, disorientation, nausea, vomiting, and constipation. Those are physical symptoms, but many dying patients suffer existential distress, including feelings of being a burden on their loved ones, meaninglessness and purposelessness, and death anxiety.

We fear being forgotten and abandoned, leaving things undone, having a life of little value, and not being missed. We fear what will happen to our loved ones without us and impoverishing our families by having a protracted death. Some patients panic about death, experience piercing remorse, have feelings of despair and worthlessness, or lose composure in the face of something terrifying and unstoppable.

Others fear the loss of dignity and privacy, soiling the bed, saying something embarrassing, being agitated, or looking ugly and pathetic. Others fear their family and friends witnessing their body and mind's intense diminishment and deterioration. What if I lose control and am judged by others? What if I need an autopsy, and my body gets mutilated? On top of all that, a bad death can be made worse by poverty, dementia, isolation, loneliness, depression, regrets, and lack of a legacy.

The Role Doctors Play

Many dying patients in today's hospitals are overtreated while their anxious loved ones are relegated to the margins and play a mainly passive role. Futile, painful, and expensive clinical interventions can continue to the end, hoping death can be defeated or postponed.

Doctors should not inflict medical procedures and tests on frail and dying patients, which may do more harm than good. Doctors are instructed through the Hippocratic oath to do no harm, but, if the dying receive excessive treatments they do not want, die in an ICU instead of at home, and die in pain and with great suffering, then isn't that harm?

The mission of doctors is to cure disease and relieve suffering. If these goals conflict at the end of life, as they often do for sick or older patients, doctors should follow the dying patient's wishes. At some point, it makes sense to cease aggressive curative care and choose palliative and hospice care instead.

Author and surgeon Atul Gawande writes in his best-selling book *Being Mortal* that textbooks used in medical school contain almost nothing on aging, frailty, or dying. He notes that many doctors know little about the realities of decline and mortality, and they understand virtually nothing about what might matter most to people as they near the end of their lives.[8]

MUCH SUFFERING IS UNNECESSARY

Dr. Ira Byock, a former professor at Dartmouth Medical School and a palliative care doctor, writes in his book *The Best Care Possible* that we make dying a lot harder than it should be, and, as a result, we are "scared to death of dying." Byock says many Americans die in hospitals or nursing homes, suffering from poorly controlled pain and other physical miseries. They often endure their final days feeling embarrassed, humiliated, lonely, confused, and a burden to others.

Prolonged serious and chronic illness, physical dependence, extreme frailty, and mental confusion are now common facts of late life. Byock reports that nearly 40 percent of people who die in a hospital spend their last days in an intensive-care unit, where they will likely be sedated or have their arms tied down so they won't pull out breathing tubes, intravenous lines, or catheters.

While acknowledging that dying is hard, he asks if it needs to be *this* hard. Byock says that the way many Americans die is a "national disgrace."[9] Go into any nursing home, for example. See the number of older women sitting in the hall outside their rooms, staring listlessly at some television drivel, or hear their unanswered cries of "Help me, please help me!" at night. We warehouse, isolate, and sequester older people in nursing homes to get them out of the way. They have no purpose or role in our communities, and we treat them like "other."

There is no universally right way for a person to die. What constitutes dying well for one person might be entirely wrong for another. The critical question is the following: How do we fully use lifesaving medical science and technology while ensuring patients are comfortable and allowed to die gently when their time comes?

HARD OR BAD DEATHS
Here are four examples of hard or bad deaths from actual cases:

1. A woman in her late eighties has been in an ICU for weeks with kidney disease, lung cancer, and diabetes. She is on a mechanical ventilator, intubated (and therefore can't talk), and on dialysis. She is miserable and knows she will never get better. The doctors keep giving her every kind of artificial life support they can think of and are still discussing a cure. The last thing this patient wanted was to die in an ICU, yoked to tubes, ventilators, and beeping machines. She wanted to die peacefully at home.

2. An older man suffers a colossal stroke that seriously damages his mind and ability to think. He doesn't recognize any loved ones, has breathing and feeding tubes, and is bedridden in an ICU. Only life support keeps him alive, but all quality of life is gone, and he is no longer the person he used to be. Unfortunately, he will likely continue in this degraded state for a long time.

3. The patient is seventy-seven years old and diagnosed with stage-4 lung cancer metastasizing to her bones and liver. She also has severe breathing issues from pneumonia. The patient said it was time for hospice. All she wanted was to go to the beach one last time and hug her four grandkids. She and her family met with her oncologist (instead of the palliative care team, who most likely would have recommended hospice), and the oncologist made it

clear that failure was not an option. He was focused on the disease and how to cure it. He "talked her into" taking the latest immuno-therapy treatment (not a cure), and the patient didn't want to dis-appoint the oncologist by "giving up." He gave her false hope. The new treatment worsened her pain and suffering, and she was robbed of precious time to talk about what mattered most to her. She never got to the beach and never enjoyed quality time with her grandkids. She likely died sooner than if she had been in hospice.[10]

4. A woman, seventy-five years old, has Alzheimer's. She watched her mother die a horrible death from Alzheimer's for more than ten years and is determined not to suffer in this way herself. In the last couple of years of her mother's life, her mother didn't recognize anyone, lay in bed in a fetal position, needed everything to be done for her, and was kept alive by life-sustaining technologies like feed-ing tubes. If this seventy-five-year-old woman doesn't take steps to avoid it, she will suffer like her mother.

Life extension should not always be the goal of health care. Physician and author Lydia Dugdale argues that far too many of us die badly.[11] In her book *The Lost Art of Dying: Reviving Forgotten Wisdom*, Dugdale contends that our reliance on modern medicine often extends suffering and stops us from dying with dignity and grace.

DOCTORS TEND TO OVERTREAT

Some estimate that up to 30 percent of medical treatment is unneces-sary.[12] Such treatment prevents us from dying peacefully and ruins the quality of the end of our lives. Toxic medications, futile surgeries, invasive tests, and other medical interventions not only cost enormous sums of money but also, especially for older patients, can have side effects that cause unnecessary harm and misery.

Overtreatment (overmedicalization) is a treatment that does more damage than it helps. Hospitals are hardwired to prolong life wherever possible, even if the costs to the patient of doing so are horrific when measured in diminished quality of life and increased pain, suffering, and separation from loved ones (because, for example, the patient is in an ICU).

As I explain more in chapter 8, you have a legal right to turn down any treatment. Just because a doctor recommends chemo, radiation, or surgery doesn't mean you have to say yes. Unless the doctor has taken the unusual step of finding out from you what matters to you and what kind of life you consider worth living, that doctor may not have any idea what you want and what your preferences are.

As the palliative care doctor, BJ Miller and his coauthor Shoshana Berger write, "In truth, saying no to a treatment can be a courageous act that frees up time and energy for all sorts of meaningful moments that might otherwise be spent distracted in a chemotherapy room, emergency department, or intensive care unit."[13]

Suppose you have dementia that has advanced to the point where you cannot recognize your friends and loved ones. You fall and break your hip. Your surgeon wants to operate, but this brings the risk of pain, potential complications, and attendant delirium associated with the operation. Your advance directive, written before you lost decision-making capability, clearly states that you want to be treated nonoperatively and with aggressive symptom management in this situation.

But your surgeon is adamant that surgery is the best course of action. These are not easy decisions, but overriding weight should be given to your wishes and goals before the onset of dementia. Only a couple of decades ago, the surgeon would automatically have gotten his way without a flicker of pushback. Thank goodness that is changing. It's hard to imagine many positive outcomes from surgery for patients with advanced dementia.

WHY DOCTORS OVERTREAT

There are several reasons why doctors tend to overtreat and overmedicalize their patients.[14]

1. Comfort care (stopping any treatment that causes pain and focusing instead on relieving suffering) is seen as "giving up." No doctors want to throw up their hands in despair and say they are out of

options. Doctors understandably dread giving bad news to their patients. To tell a patient that, for example, chemotherapy is no longer effective or helpful is agonizing. It is easier to keep offering treatments, however fruitless. To take advantage of hospice, a patient has to give up curative treatment, so comfort care is easily interpreted as "giving up." In addition, many doctors don't like discussing dying and death with their patients. Ordering more tests and treatments is much easier than talking about end-of-life issues.

2. Many patients and their loved ones never want to give up fighting for life either. The pressure from families on doctors to keep treating, and thus impose pain and suffering on their dying loved one, can be immense. When families pressure doctors to "do anything they can" to save the life of an older loved one, they often do not realize the torture that this will inflict on the patient. Families are terrified of losing their beloved nana or grandpa and try to avoid the pain of their grief by telling doctors to "do everything." But accepting a gentle and swift death is better than imposing ineffective and painful treatments that gain a few days of life but at the cost of a horrific quality of life.

3. Doctors fear malpractice lawsuits and are inclined to practice "defensive medicine." Doctors would rather order unnecessary tests and treatments than risk being sued by devastated and fraught loved ones of patients who have died.

4. When hospitals acquire fancy, cutting-edge medical technology, it brings understandable pressure to use it. Doctors may also believe that applying a treatment, especially one that is new and unproven, could lead to new knowledge that might help future patients.

5. Doctors receive payment for conducting tests and treatments like surgeries and are financially rewarded for doing more rather than doing better. Aggressive interventions are more profitable and lucrative than measures (e.g., given by geriatricians and palliative care doctors) that help older patients have a better quality of life.

Dr. Richard Stuart, psychologist and professor emeritus in the University of Washington's Department of Psychiatry, writes,

> Patients often unwittingly consent to this escalation of care. Often, without formally articulating the policy, almost all health-care organizations ask patients to rapidly sign detailed, small-print consent forms through which they accept unqualified use of resuscitation, as well as other, often unspecified interventions. Unfortunately, the traditional treatments these documents warrant are often not concordant with the intervention patients thought they were agreeing to accept.[15]

OVERMEDICALIZATION

Aggressive overmedicalization is associated with a worse patient quality of life. Numerous large studies published in peer-reviewed journals have shown that patients who receive extensive medical interventions (such as intensive care and ventilators) at the end of life have zero life extension and often more discomfort than those who choose hospice care and die at home surrounded by their families.[16]

Imagine an aggressive treatment that would give you a few extra weeks of life. That sounds like a good deal, but what if those few additional weeks of life are marked by severe nausea and having to be in intensive care attached to many uncomfortable tubes and machines? Are those few weeks worth it, especially if you prize being free of pain, having autonomy, living at home, engaging in affectionate conversations with loved ones, and not imposing financial and other burdens on family members? The gung-ho doctor who wants you to have the treatment may only have the goal of keeping you alive no matter the cost in pain, suffering, and loss of quality of life.

IS SURGERY IN OLDER PATIENTS ALWAYS A BAD IDEA?

The answer is no. With proper planning, says former Maryland state legislator, author, and emergency-medicine physician Dan Morhaim, surgery for seniors can go well, but surgeons need to be careful about and sensitive to the needs of their patients.[17] The best approach depends on the specifics of the case and the preferences of the patient. In his book

Preparing for a Better End, Morhaim says obtaining a second and even a third opinion is always wise.[18]

Even if surgery on older patients isn't always a bad idea, it is best to be skeptical and wary. *In Knocking on Heaven's Door*, author Katy Butler vividly describes her frustrating and unsuccessful effort to deactivate her father's pacemaker as he sank into dementia and frailty. Her book shows how doctors want to treat patients with medical interventions even when they are not warranted or justified. Butler's family was overwhelmed by a cavalcade of treatments her father might have been better off without.[19]

Nursing PhD student Lila Moersch showed through her research that hospitalization for older patients leads to decreased mobility because of muscle deconditioning. After only a week, older adults can lose so much muscle mass that they can't take care of themselves. They can't walk, and they can't shower. Hospitals are not good places for older people, even if the hospital stays are short.[20]

"Post-hospital syndrome" is real and probably underlies the stubbornly high rate of hospital readmissions among older patients.[21] The stress of hospitalization can increase a patient's vulnerability to a range of other health problems. Geriatrician and researcher Kenneth Covinsky at the University of California at San Francisco found that one-third of patients seventy and older leave the hospital more disabled than when they arrived.[22]

As Dr. Sam Harrington writes in his book *At Peace: Choosing a Good Death after a Long Life*, the health-care system in America wasn't designed to treat the aging population with care and compassion. Many older patients die in institutions such as hospitals and nursing homes when they would rather die at home. Many undergo painful procedures at the end of their lives instead of having a peaceful death.[23]

Dr. Lydia Dugdale raises this question in her book *The Lost Art of Dying*: At what point should we stop going to the hospital? She points out that it's more complex than age because people vary so much, with some ninety-year-olds being robust and vigorous while some seventy-year-olds are frail and weak. The bottom line for Dugdale is that frail people—those who walk very slowly, have low physical activity, have a weak handgrip, feel constantly fatigued and exhausted, and are losing weight unintentionally—should avoid a hospital if possible.[24]

Dugdale's conclusion is supported by many studies that show older and frail patients do not thrive in hospitals.[25] They suffer more complications and are more negatively affected by the stresses that naturally come with a hospital stay (such as unhealthy food, inactivity, noise, and interrupted sleep) as well as the risk of getting even sicker from hospital-generated infections. Beyond that, being in a hospital is a generally disagreeable experience; one is without the comforts of home, surrounded by the unfamiliar and sterile, and subject to the medical staff's often confusing rules, practices, and quirks.

CARDIOPULMONARY RESUSCITATION FOR OLDER PATIENTS

Cardiopulmonary resuscitation (CPR) is an effort by doctors and nurses to revive patients after they have stopped breathing or their heart has stopped. Medical providers typically use powerful pushes on the chest together with shocking the heart with a defibrillator. This makes a lot of sense on a strong person, but when CPR is applied to the frail, old, and the terminally ill, it can be futile and harmful because survival rates are very low.

In the absence of a medical directive, such as a physician order for life-sustaining treatment (POLST, see chapter 4), a hospital will give patients CPR, even if the patients are in their nineties or have an advanced illness, because the mission of a hospital is to save lives, and applying CPR is a standard operating procedure. But using CPR close to the end of life means, with near certainty, that a peaceful death for the patient becomes virtually impossible. And the likelihood of surviving resuscitation for chronically ill older patients is tiny.

Author and hospice chaplain Hank Dunn writes that, today, in hospitals, nursing homes, and residential care facilities, "CPR has become standard practice on all patients who experience heart or breathing failure, except for those with orders restricting its use."[26] These restricting orders go by different names, including DNR (do not resuscitate), DNAR (do not attempt resuscitation), AND (allow natural death), No Code, or No CPR.

If a patient's heart stops in a hospital, a "code" is called, and the patient is likely to experience CPR, injection of medications, and mechanical ventilation. CPR and these other treatments significantly reduce the chances of the patient having a peaceful death.[27] Dunn says, "Often the most loving thing to do (for older and very sick patients) is to let loved ones die in peace without the aggressiveness of CPR."[28]

The CPR we see on television in high-intensity medical dramas often gives a misleading notion of its effectiveness. We see sick people quickly returning to good health after receiving CPR. Doctors and nurses in *ER* and *Grey's Anatomy* save more than 75 percent of their patients. The truth is that CPR is rarely successful, especially for older people.[29] Dugdale says that only about 10 to 20 percent of resuscitated patients survive to leave the hospital.[30]

Similarly, emergency-medicine physician Dan Morhaim says CPR is rarely effective. He points out that survival rates from CPR, when started in a community setting, average about 5 percent and a little above that in a hospital setting.[31] Morhaim says CPR has its place, but, for patients who are unlikely to benefit from it, it is "closer to torture than healing."[32] Similarly, Dr. Sam Harrington writes, "CPR is much more brutal and much less effective than people are led to believe. . . . When the patient is old, infirm, or suffering from a terminal illness, [using CPR] is cruel and reflects poor judgment."[33] Of the few older patients who are revived by CPR after suffering a cardiac arrest at home, fewer than 2 percent live for one month.[34]

Doing a "full code" on an older, dying person, in which the patient is pounded, shocked, and intubated (a tube forced down the patient's throat to supply air), allows doctors to tell the patient's loved ones, "We did everything possible to save her." However, the patient has just experienced the most brutal and painful death. Many doctors realize that "code" activity on an older person is often more like torture than care. It produces misery and suffering, and—even if a few days of life are gained—the quality of life is severely compromised.

ICUS AND OLDER PATIENTS

From 30 to 40 percent of patients have an ICU admission in the last month of life. Nine out of ten people with profound dementia have some invasive procedure in the last month of life. Most of these health expenditures are wasteful and should be stopped for humane and compassionate reasons. An ICU is well-known for reviving and giving life to patients who would otherwise die, especially after a car accident or an acute illness. But, for older people, going to an ICU may not always be wise.

Sometimes, a patient near the end of life will want to choose comfort care over painful, life-prolonging treatments. As the Hippocratic oath says, "Warmth, sympathy, and understanding may outweigh the surgeon's knife or the chemist's drug."[35]

Before Dr. Jessica Zitter became a palliative care doctor, she was an ICU doctor, and she admits that, as an ICU doctor, it was easy to demean and "objectify" her patients. She writes, "This denial is particularly easy in the ICU. My patients were often comatose, tied down, and sedated. I never had the chance to get to know them as the people they had been, their histories, personalities, and quirks."[36]

ICUs encourage mechanized and painful deaths where patients are separated from their families and in a scary, cold environment. In her valiant efforts to save lives, Zitter realized she often worsened the dying process. She also hadn't realized how prevalent pain was in the ICU and how much suffering patients were experiencing.[37] Shockingly, more than 50 percent of Americans die in pain.[38]

It typically does not make sense to place older and critically ill patients suffering from geriatric conditions such as disability, frailty, multimorbidity, and dementia in the ICU. They are unlikely to benefit from it. For an older patient with, say, metastatic cancer and not long to live, ICU interventions such as electric shocks, chest compressions, and mechanical ventilation are inappropriate and only serve to guarantee a bad death. It is far better to die peacefully in hospice at home with comfort care and excellent pain management.

It's not true that ICUs are *never* appropriate for older people. If a vigorous and vibrant ninety-year-old gets pneumonia or a urinary-tract infection, then time in an ICU may be precisely what is needed, and the

ICU can add value to life. However, going into an ICU increases the probability that the patient will end up with a prolonged and miserable death.[39] Also, remember that many families can be traumatized by witnessing the terrible deterioration and pain their loved ones suffer in ICUs, where doctors focus on keeping patients alive regardless of their quality of life.

MORAL DISTRESS SUFFERED BY MEDICAL PROVIDERS WORKING IN ICUS

Doctors and nurses called to a full code for the frail aging often suffer what is called "moral distress" when they want to allow a natural, peaceful death but then are forced to use electric defibrillators to shock the heart and powerful thrusting on the chest (often cracking ribs). The hospital rules and protocols demand that they "do everything" to keep the patient alive.

"Moral distress" is the emotional pain of medical providers forced to do something to patients that violates their moral values. It's often used to describe the torment of doctors and nurses working in an ICU caring for patients who are dying painfully, partly because of medical treatments they have received in the ICU.

Artificially prolonging lives that should not be prolonged and are consumed with pain and suffering gives medical providers moral distress because the doctors and nurses feel they are hurting rather than helping. The purpose of health care should not be to prolong life at all costs. Because some treatment is good, it doesn't mean more treatment is better.

HOW LONELINESS AND ISOLATION CAN WORSEN DYING

People are more likely to have a good death if they are part of a community, so it is essential to make it a priority to build relationships throughout our lives. Loneliness can make a good death hard to achieve. Psychiatrist Irvin Yalom describes loneliness as "greatly increasing the anguish of dying."[40] Anything we can do to help the dying person feel less lonely and more part of a community (like a family) will be helpful. Dying separates us not only from our loved ones but also from the world itself and all our unique memories.

Frequently, our death-denying society makes those who are dying feel isolated. Friends and loved ones become more distant because they fear saying the wrong thing and distressing the person near death. They may also hang back because getting too close brings them face-to-face with their own terrifying death. The dying may be complicit and may even encourage their loneliness because they know that isolation and silence can help protect their caregivers and loved ones from awkwardness and discomfort.

Sometimes the dying process can make people less pleasant to be around (e.g., they smell or get cranky). That feeds into older people's isolation and creates a negative feedback loop, making them even more unpleasant to be around. As a result, the goal of being included, respected, and loved becomes elusive, exacerbated by our society's unfriendly attitude toward older people.

Few experiences can be more awful than dying in an understaffed nursing home with underpaid, fatigued, and overworked nursing staff when you are lonely, bedridden, have bedsores, are incontinent of bladder and stool, and are tube-fed or spoon-fed. It is hard to have a good death under such circumstances. Barbara Karnes, RN, writes, "Dying is not a medical event. It is a social, communal event, and, most importantly, it is a natural event. It is the body doing what it is naturally programmed to do. We can ease its transition by keeping it as comfortable as we can."[41]

How Doctors Want to Die

We can gain insight into what makes a good death by observing what doctors do when they die. Doctors frequently see dying patients and know better than most people what makes a good death. What doctors want to do at the end of their lives is revealing. In November 2011, a retired family doctor in Los Angeles, Ken Murray, published an article entitled "How Doctors Die."[42] Murray pointed out that doctors behave differently at the end of their lives than most people. They have fewer aggressive interventions, suffer less, and take advantage of palliative care, including hospice.

They eschew the harsh treatments (such as surgeries, radiation, and chemotherapy) they regularly hand out to their older patients. Typically, doctors will stop treatment, refuse CPR, take painkillers as appropriate, and be surrounded by loved ones at home. What's unusual about doctors is not how much treatment they get compared with most Americans but how little. As a result, they tend to die gently.

Dr. VJ Periyakoil at Stanford University published research in 2014 showing that nearly nine in ten doctors said they would choose a DNR status when dying. Yet often doctors do not offer that option to their patients.[43] Further studies have shown that doctors are likelier to die at home and spend less time in an ICU.[44]

Medical technology can stop people from dying, but it can also rob life from the dying. ICU and palliative care physician Dr. Jessica Zitter writes,

> I would not want a breathing tube thrust down my throat or to be the recipient of cardiac resuscitation if I am in the final stages of a terminal or life-limiting disease, even with all of my faculties present. I don't want to have my arms, legs, and airway tied to a bed for my final days or even weeks. I would not want large catheters threaded into my neck or groin to deliver dialysis if I were on the verge of death. These things happen all the time, and I won't have it for myself.[45]

Similarly, palliative care and hospice physician Dr. Sunita Puri writes, "Most physicians I knew noticed the irony inherent in our offering patients intubations, CPR, tracheostomies, dialysis, and so on, when many of us wouldn't choose such interventions for ourselves in their circumstances."[46] And emergency-room doctor Dan Morhaim writes, "We have to end the disconnect between what doctors want for themselves and what we (doctors) offer to patients."[47]

Cardiologist Dr. Haider Warraich says that most doctors value the quality of their life far more than its length. Doctors rarely want to have CPR performed on them if the need arises.[48] Doctors know things that patients may not know but should be told. For example, chemotherapy for older patients can be incredibly taxing and arduous. It can cause nausea, vomiting, depression, mouth sores, sore muscles, and brain fog. It can also weaken the heart and damage the kidneys. Chemo can make one's last days unbearably painful.[49]

Dr. BJ Miller and Shoshana Berger write, "If you know you are going to die someday from (an) incurable illness, are in an advanced stage, and seek a peaceful or comfortable death, we unequivocally recommend your code status be DNR."[50]

One way to close the gap between patients and doctors concerning dying well is to make patients more informed. After all, it's because doctors are more knowledgeable about what happens at the end of life that they can make better decisions. We can inform patients by taking them on tours of the ICU. Another approach is to educate patients about sophisticated medical treatments by showing them videos of what happens. Perhaps patients would have second thoughts about ventilation or feeding tubes (percutaneous endoscopic gastrostomy [PEG] tubes) if they could see the reality.[51]

DOCTORS DON'T ALWAYS KNOW WHAT IS BEST FOR THEIR PATIENTS

Barbara Coombs Lee points out that an overwhelming majority of Americans (71 percent) believe improving the quality of life for seriously ill patients is more important, even if it means a shorter life.[52] More and more patients, especially older patients, realize they can say no to potentially harmful treatments, including breathing machines (trach tubes), PEG tubes, cardiac resuscitation with electric shocks and chest compressions (CPR), and dialysis.

ICU doctor Dr. Jessica Zitter writes, "CPR is often of no real benefit for many of the patients upon whom we use it, and feeding tubes can actually be harmful for many."[53] She adds that "these facts are widely unknown, even by some of the physicians who administer these procedures."[54]

SLOW MEDICINE

One way to increase our chances of achieving a good death is to be treated by doctors who believe in and practice "slow medicine." Slow medicine is an international movement started in Italy to reform medicine. At its core is the notion that doctors should take the time to consider the needs of the whole patient, make a thorough and careful diagnosis, and form a trusting and healing relationship with the patient. Slow medicine believes that to do more is not necessarily to do better. Tests and treatments should not be hastily prescribed.

Medical schools tend to produce doctors who are schooled in "fast medicine," meaning they are skilled at putting patients on what Dr. Jessica Zitter calls "a conveyor belt" that moves speedily through invasive tests, surgery, CPR, chemo, and whatever other aggressive tests and treatments are available.

Two doctors who pioneered slow medicine in the United States are Dr. Dennis McCullough, author of *My Mother, Your Mother*, and Dr. Victoria Sweet, author of *Slow Medicine*. Good examples of slow medicine are hospice, palliative, and comfort care. "Fast medicine" tends to optimize the well-being of doctors rather than of patients. This is wrong. We must optimize the health and well-being of the patient, not the needs, goals, and desires of the hospital or doctor.

Sweet argues that, in fast medicine, doctors give little thought to the patient as a whole because they fixate on a particular organ, such as the liver or heart.[55] Older people, in particular, need "slow medicine," a more thoughtful, intentional, compassionate approach to medicine, where the whole person, not just a disease or an organ, is considered.

Slow medicine is often ideal for older patients suffering from comorbidities (several illnesses simultaneously). It lessens the risk of medical interventions occurring with deadly side effects. Science writer and end-of-life expert Katy Butler writes, "The older or frailer we get, the wider the gap is likely to grow between the treatments fast medicine offers and the thoughtful, time-consuming, gentle, coordinated care we need most."[56]

FAST MEDICINE CAN POSE RISKS TO OLDER PATIENTS

Is it a good idea to give antibiotics for pneumonia (once called "the old man's friend") to frail patients in their nineties who are terminally ill with, say, cancer and are near death? Pneumonia may be a gentler, more peaceful way to die than painful cancer.

Fast medicine can pose risks to older patients who may be frail and have comorbidities caused by multiple factors and not easily solved by one dramatic treatment or drug. Poor digestion, constipation, nausea, vertigo, poor sleep, melancholy, pain, and too many pills with harmful side effects require a thoughtful, collaborative, patient-directed approach by medical providers.

Not enough patients near the end of their lives are given information about slow medicine or about the benefits of palliative care, hospice, comfort care, and no treatment. Too many patients misinterpret the word "treatment" to mean "cure," when all the doctor may mean is that it may extend the patient's life by a few weeks and at the cost of intense discomfort.

There is no "correct" or "incorrect" decision at the end of life. The only thing that matters is that any decision be patient-directed (more on that below) and what the patient wants. One patient may wish to be intubated, have CPR, and have mechanical ventilation. Another might feel that artificial ventilation is a terrible experience for an older person (and for their loved ones to have to see). That patient may prefer to ask for morphine to alleviate any sense of air hunger and to allow a gentle death.

Having a breathing tube down your throat is a horrible experience, as I can testify from firsthand experience. Patients often fight and flail against the intense discomfort and must be tied down or even sedated to tolerate the intubation. Of course, they can't speak, so the overall effect on patients and their families is highly distressing.

Slow medicine brings a more thoughtful approach to caring for patients. It means the doctor deeply understands the patient, is kind and thoughtful, does not rush into harsh treatments, and communicates clearly and candidly. Slow medicine might result in an elderly, frail person saying no to an aggressive intervention, such as surgery, and instead deciding to focus on preserving as high a quality of life as possible for as long as possible.

COMFORT CARE

The best way to understand comfort care is to contrast it with seeking a cure or life-sustaining care. Life-sustaining care is keeping a patient (who may be unconscious or cognitively impaired) alive with advanced medical procedures, artificial feeding, and mechanical ventilation. Comfort care focuses not on extending life, regardless of quality, but on improving the quality of the patient's life.

If you have a terminal disease, then a cure is extremely unlikely. Life-sustaining treatments may keep your heart, lungs, and other organs working, but your quality of life, as measured by interactions with others, cognitive awareness, ability to move, etc., may be minimal. That said, deciding when to seek comfort care and stop pursuing a cure or life-sustaining care can be fraught and complicated.

PATIENT-DIRECTED CARE

One characteristic of slow medicine is patient-directed care. This happens when patients work closely with their doctors to select treatments and tests that align with their priorities and values. Under these favorable circumstances, patients understand their illness and the prognosis and outcomes. They also understand the various treatment options, including the option of no treatment and the pros and cons of each treatment being considered. All the doctor has to do is be honest, realistic, and informed, and, above all, listen to the patient.

Sadly, ICU and palliative care physician Dr. Jessica Zitter says that shared decision-making "rarely occurs" and that "too many critically important decisions are made for patients without their input when they are no longer able to voice their preferences."[57] Three reasons this occurs are our fear of death and unwillingness to talk about it, medical schools that fail to train doctors on how to have these conversations, and a medical system that inadequately compensates doctors for using patient-directed care.

Patient-directed care is a much-needed reform movement whose mission is to make the patient's needs, rather than those of insurance companies, health-care systems, and medical-care providers, the driving force for medical decision-making and care.

DO NOT PUT BLIND FAITH IN DOCTORS

Many doctors assume they know what's best for the patient. But we need to redefine the doctor-patient relationship. *New York Times* columnist Frank Bruni writes in his memoir *The Beauty of Dusk,*

> Doctors are flawed. They're human. We want them to be gods, because we want that certainty, that salvation. We want clear roles: The doctor commands; the patient obeys. But, at times, in their imperfection and arrogance and haste, they make assumptions and mistakes. So it's crucial to approach a relationship with a doctor, any doctor, as a partnership and to consider yourself an equal partner, respectful but not obsequious, receptive but skeptical.[58]

We should not place blind faith in doctors and should never be intimidated by them. So many patients think, "My doctor will know what is best for me." This opinion must be respected, and confidence in doctors is positive. However, the brutal truth is that medical providers don't always know what is best. This is especially true when they have not bothered to get to know their patients and learn what is truly important to them.

Doctors sometimes think they know the right thing to do, regardless of what anyone else thinks or what is written in the patient's advance directive. These doctors find the term "patient-directed care" puzzling and even unappealing. Palliative care physician Dr. Sunita Puri writes, "We (doctors) cannot fix everything. In fact, we can only slow down rather than cure most debilitating chronic diseases, maladies including heart failure and emphysema and multiple sclerosis, all of which slowly progress, claiming our lives."[59]

THE JOB OF DOCTORS IS TO RELIEVE SUFFERING

People die badly because many well-intentioned doctors want to keep us alive as long as possible. Medical schools teach doctors that the longer patients live, the more successful they are. But more and more doctors, led by palliative care and hospice doctors, are realizing that their job is to relieve suffering, and they are failing to relieve suffering when they perform futile and aggressive medical interventions near the end of life. Such interventions may add a few days or weeks of life, but they also destroy any quality of life and often seem more like torture than health care.

Doctors are experts on disease or a particular organ, like the heart or liver, but they are not experts on the patient. Dr. Jessica Zitter says, "They may know what to do *to* the patient but know little about what to do *for* the patient." Of course, some doctors will say, "Our job is to keep people alive as long as possible," but doctors should remind themselves of their most important task: to reduce suffering and to do what the patient wants, not what the doctor wants.

* * * * *

This chapter has defined and described a good death. In the next chapter, we will focus on how to live well so as to die well.

CHAPTER 2

Live Well to Die Well

Having a good death is not simply a question of luck. Intentionality plays a significant role in how well we die. To live well is to get ready to die well. Our daily lives create the person we will be when we die and, thus, the kind of death we will experience. This chapter explores how the way we live shapes the way we die. As nurse and author Sallie Tisdale writes, "With every passing day, we create the kind of death we will have."[1]

Ars Moriendi

The idea that in order to die well you have to live well goes back hundreds of years. In the fourteenth century, when so many priests died from the bubonic plague that there were not enough priests to care for the dying, a book called *Ars Moriendi* (the "art of dying") described how people could prepare for death without needing a priest. Dr. Lydia Dugdale describes *Ars Moriendi* in her book *The Lost Art of Dying*.[2] *Ars Moriendi* encourages readers to think about how they live, how they die, how to prepare for death, and how to die well. In addition, the rules of *Ars Moriendi* provide practical guidance for the dying and their caregivers.

The central theme of *Ars Moriendi* is that, to have a good death, we have to live well. We must admit we are going to die at some point and that, in the meantime, while we still have blood pumping through our bodies, we are going to work out our purpose in life and why our relationships with others are so important.

35

PEOPLE DIE THE WAY THEY LIVE

It's common knowledge among hospice nurses that, more often than not, people die as they have lived. Angry people in life tend to die angrily and unhappily. Kind, gentle people tend to die peacefully. It rarely happens that rancorous, vitriolic people become patient and thoughtful on their deathbed, or people who are kind and generous in life turn into selfish monsters as they die.

After watching his beloved mother die, psychiatrist Dr. Barry Gorman says, "The patient's demeanor also has an effect on those around them and affects the whole atmosphere of the room."[3] A confident and prepared individual can calm those around him or her and make it possible for them to be fully present and to grieve.

The more intentional our life is, the more likely we will die well. Intentional people pursue what matters to them and live a life of meaning, purpose, and joy. They overcome setbacks and failures, stay focused on their goals, and die with few regrets.[4] An intentional and successful life has little to do with wealth, income, social status, or possessions. It involves living fully and with intention. End-of-life expert and author Katy Butler writes in her book *The Art of Dying Well*, "People who are willing to contemplate their aging, vulnerability, and mortality often live better lives in old age and illness, and experience better deaths, than those who don't."[5]

WHY PLANNING AND PREPARING FOR A GOOD DEATH IS IMPORTANT

People are understandably fearful of death because it's a big unknown. It means the end of our relationship with those we love and cherish. We tend not to prepare for death because we are afraid and think dying doesn't apply to us. Or we think we are encouraging death by thinking about it. Dying is the last thing we want to think about and plan for. However, if we plan and prepare, we can die better, with fewer regrets, less pain, less suffering, and less trauma for those who love us and witness our last days.

If we don't plan and prepare, we may die without completing the five life tasks that palliative care doctor Ira Byock recommends we all need to do: expressing love, thanking, forgiving, being forgiven, and saying goodbye. Without preparation and planning, your caregivers (soon to be your survivors) may not know whether to inform you that you are dying, what type of medical care you want, whether you want to be cremated or embalmed, and what kind of memorial service you would like. Their ignorance of those things will exacerbate their grief and stress.

If you want a good death, you must start planning for it before you are on your deathbed. While you are healthy, consider the end of your life.

Memento Mori

A key element of planning and preparation is acknowledging that we will die. Some people keep a memento mori (such as a small plastic model of a human skull) nearby to remind them that death is unavoidable and that we should not fear or hide from it. A beneficial Buddhist practice is to imagine your own death. The grief and sadness, the unfinished projects, everything you would miss, your partner remarrying, grandchildren not knowing you, the fond words you would say to your loved ones and friends, and so on. Can you fully accept that you will die and the world will continue without you? When practicing Buddhists wake up each morning, they reflect on death so they do not take life for granted and are grateful that they are alive for another day.

Getting Older Doesn't Mean You Are Dying

For most people, being an older person and the process of dying are inextricably linked, but this is wrong. Here are four myths about being older.

1. Older age is a problem and full of suffering and stress. Wrong! Geriatricians will tell you that most older people are active, happy, and fully engaged in all kinds of exciting projects.[6]

2. Older age is a breeze if you have money and your health. Wrong again! The famous longitudinal Harvard study shows that *relationships* are the key to happiness and fulfillment.[7]

3. Younger is always better, and getting old means becoming irrelevant and useless. Wrong again! Many studies have shown that from

childhood onward, happiness declines and then dramatically rises. Happiness in older age typically far exceeds happiness at age forty. Aging results in better emotional regulation, more compassion and equanimity, more profound gratitude, and more engagement with the present.[8]

4. Illness and disease are inevitable parts of aging. Nope! The Mayo Clinic says health problems commonly attributed to aging are due to inactivity, unhealthy diets, smoking, or other lifestyle choices.[9] The American Cancer Society (ACS) says more than half of all cancer deaths could be prevented if Americans took better care of themselves.[10] In other words, we can delay the onset of disease and increase our health span—the number of years we are healthy—through better lifestyle choices.

Growing older can potentially be so much more than growing old. It's a time to thrive in new ways, and, the more we thrive, the more likely we are to achieve a good death.

OLD-OLD AGE VERSUS YOUNG-OLD AGE[11]

Let's not pretend that being older brings with it no challenges. Old age *is* a problem if you are referring to *old-old* age. Old-old age can be challenging and distressing, and we shouldn't whitewash it. Most of us strive to delay the onset of old-old age as long as possible. Physical pain, loss of autonomy, an inability to read or hear, increasing disintegration, chronic and sudden indignities, depression, poorly run nursing homes, overmedicalization, and so on are all scary and alarming. Psychoanalyst Erik Erikson calls this final stage of life "the ninth stage" in his life-cycle theory.[12] It's the time when debility and suffering have the upper hand. In the ninth stage, advance directives, do-not-resuscitate orders, palliative care, and hospice are vital.

But *young-old age*—the period of old age *before* we suffer from significant impairment—starts at about sixty or sixty-five and can go on for many years if we take good care of ourselves. This is the period in our lives which, if we live wisely, can significantly impact the quality of our dying and death. According to the Pew Charitable Trust, only 25 percent of aging is genetic, while 75 percent is environmental and lifestyle, including diet, exercise, relationships, stress, and smoking.[13] Getting older doesn't necessarily mean deterioration. Erikson's ninth stage starts later than it used to because our health spans are getting longer.

Growth at the End of Life

As we age, we can develop personally and exercise wisdom, purpose, and creativity. We can build a legacy for our children and the next generation. All this will increase our chances of experiencing a good death. Aging is not to be dreaded but embraced because it brings new opportunities. We can do so much more than merely survive. It is an opportunity for growth. And if we seek opportunities to grow, we are more likely to feel fulfilled and die well.[14]

What does your ideal older age or elderhood look like? How will you find meaning and purpose as an older person? What is the vision you have for yourself as you grow older? One way of creating this vision is to produce a personal mission statement. A personal mission statement describes what matters to you, your values, the kind of person you want to be, and what you'd like to accomplish before you die. It is critical to living an intentional life.[15]

Here are two examples of personal mission statements, even if the authors didn't necessarily call them by that name. Arthur Conan Doyle wrote, "I should dearly love that the world should be ever so little better for my presence and that I throw all my weight on the scale of tolerance, charity, temperance, peace, and kindliness." And George Bernard Shaw famously wrote, "Life is no 'brief candle' to me. It is a sort of splendid torch, which I have got hold of for a moment, and I want to make it burn as brightly as possible before handing it on to future generations." A personal mission statement—a vision for your life—will help you have a better death.

Imagining Your Own Funeral

Here is one way to create a personal mission statement. Imagine you're entering a big building. As you open the door and look inside, you see one to two hundred people with their backs to you. You strain to see what they are looking at. And then you spot it. They're looking at a casket, and you suddenly realize you're witnessing a funeral. As you try to fathom what's happening, you see a person you know well and who loves you standing up to give a eulogy. You realize, with great fascination, that you are witnessing your own funeral.

What do you want to hear said about you? As you think about this, assume you've led an honorable and successful life. What are the assessments you would like the eulogist to make about you? What character traits and behaviors would you like the person to praise and be grateful for? What have you accomplished? Were you compassionate, kind, and generous? What kind of friend or family member were you? What were your values?

Answering these questions will help you flesh out your personal mission statement, and doing that will help you live an abundant, full life. *New York Times* columnist David Brooks discusses the distinction between resume and eulogy virtues.[16] Resumé virtues are the strengths you put on your work bio. For example, the ability to prosecute, sell houses, or help others with their taxes. But when you are on your deathbed, most people are not thinking of resumé virtues. Instead, they are thinking of eulogy virtues. How well do you love your family? Did you show empathy, charity, and openhandedness? What kind of character did you develop? Did you have integrity? At the end of your life, these questions loom large. You are imagining your best possible future self.[17]

The author Katherine Mansfield writes, "If you wish to live, you must first attend your own funeral." What she means by this paradox is, to live well, you should think ahead to your funeral and ask what will be said in your eulogy. What will you have accomplished in your life? And what will those closest to you say about your character?

COMPOSE A PERSONAL MISSION STATEMENT

Imagining your own funeral reflects the wisdom of one of Steven R. Covey's habits, as described in his 1989 book *The Seven Habits of Highly Effective People*: "Begin with the end in mind." What do you want your life as an older person to look like? Unfortunately, few of us think about this question. As teenagers and young adults, we think about and plan our futures, but, as we get older, we tend to stop thinking about how to become our best future selves. This is a mistake. Whether young or old, having a personal mission statement (a vision for your life) is essential. Whatever age you are, you need a life full of meaning and purpose.[18] This can be crucial to achieving a good death.

We must compose a personal mission statement to increase our chances of having a good dying experience and a good death. It doesn't have to be perfect. It's constantly evolving and is a work in progress like each of us. Having a vision for our life and spelling out in writing our life goals as part of that vision can give us not only a good death but also energy and purpose, especially when facing challenges, such as feeling anxious, sleeping poorly, feeling disconnected from loved ones, feeling in a rut, or worrying about pandemics.[19]

As we design our personal mission statement, we should be ambitious and craft a document that excites and inspires us. In doing so, we are crafting and shaping ourselves into a generous, wise, purposeful, and creative person who is more likely to make choices that will help us die well. Dr. Lydia Dugdale, a doctor and medical ethicist, writes, "If we live deliberately, with gratitude and with attention to what matters most, our lives will be richer and our dying better."[20]

ORGANIZE LIFE GOALS

One way to organize life goals in a personal mission statement is to group them according to the four fundamental dimensions of our nature: physical, social/emotional, mental, spiritual.

Physical includes exercise, diet, and sleep. As you know, moving our body daily, eating lots of fruits and vegetables, and getting sound sleep are all critical. Remember that some seventy-year-olds are healthier than a sedentary thirty-five-year-old. A shocking fact is that more than 80 million Americans over the age of six are entirely inactive.[21]

Social/emotional includes love, friendship, and community. One goal to consider in this area is writing a "gratitude" letter. This is a heartfelt letter to those you love, thanking them for their love and caring. You tell them what they mean to you. You tell them you love them. You tell them what you appreciate about them. Receiving a letter like that is deeply meaningful. (More on ideas like this, including legacy letters and ethical wills, can be found in chapter 5.)

Mental includes learning, studying, and reading. One goal to consider in this area is writing a memoir. It doesn't have to be lengthy. It would be part of your legacy, a gift to future generations who want to know about your successes, setbacks, and struggles. As the African proverb says, a library burns to the ground when an older person dies. We need to preserve each of our "libraries." (More on memoirs can be found in chapter 5.)

Spiritual includes finding a purpose and meaning in our lives. Geriatricians will tell you they see stunning revitalization in older people when a newfound purpose comes along.[22] One goal to consider in this area is to keep a gratitude journal, a thoughtful chronicling of the things we are grateful for. A gratitude journal is an instrument of self-awareness to help us savor what is going well in our lives.

Setting challenging goals for ourselves in each of those four dimensions is vital. These goals should advance the values and vision in our personal mission statement. This will help us live well, and we are more likely to die well if we live well. Setting goals is the best way to find purpose and meaning in life and to give us a reason to live.[23] Having inspiring goals and living a life of worth will help us have the fewest regrets at the end of life.

OLDER PEOPLE ARE CHANGING

Older people across America are using their later years to create new lives. They're trying new careers, volunteering, returning to school, making new friends, creating villages (more on villages below), and pursuing new interests. People like Jane Goodall, Jane Fonda, Condoleezza Rice, Mick Jagger, Paul McCartney, and Gloria Steinem are redefining what it means to be old. Older people are thinking hard about what matters and spending more time on the relationships, causes, and goals they care deeply about.

We need to be more ambitious and intentional when thinking about the end of our lives and not leave it to chance. We need to be less haphazard. In her book *Elderhood*, Dr. Louise Aronson, a geriatric-care doctor, writes, "We desperately want our elderhood to be long, meaningful, and satisfying, yet most of us refuse to approach it with the same shameless ambition we reflexively accord childhood and adulthood."[24]

THE INSIDIOUS NATURE OF AGEISM

When I was younger, I associated old age with deterioration, disease, and frailty. Older folks seemed to be limping pitifully toward their deaths. I realize now I was being ageist (seeing aging as a time of decay), one of the obstacles to living a full and intentional life and achieving a good death. Psychologist Dr. Becca Levy at Yale University has shown that ageism inflicts far more damage than one might think. It can shorten people's lives and damage their cognitive and physical health.[25]

Dr. Levy's 2002 longevity study followed hundreds of older residents in an Ohio town for two decades and found—amazingly—that people lived seven and a half years longer if they had positive beliefs about aging compared to those with the most negative attitudes.[26] People who embrace harmful stereotypes of older people put themselves at risk of poor health and early death.[27]

When we denigrate and stigmatize older people, even unconsciously, we devalue our future selves. Devaluing older people is to belittle and be biased against the person we will become. Demonizing old age reduces health spans, and an early, premature death cannot be considered a good death, however peaceful. A life shackled and restricted by ageism makes a good death impossible.

Ageism is a prejudice still widely sanctioned in society. Growing older is the butt of demeaning jokes. Older people are not considered for jobs for which they are qualified. Marketers and advertisers crave what is young and new. As a result, older people often feel invisible and ignored despite their wisdom, energy, skills, and rich experiences.[28]

Dr. Robert N. Butler, a pioneering gerontologist, psychiatrist, and founding director of the National Institute of Aging[29], created the term "ageism" in the 1970s to describe discrimination against older people and negatively stereotyping them. He wrote, "We subtly cease to identify with them as human beings, which enables us to feel more comfortable about our neglect and dislike of them."[30]

At first glance, ageism may not seem to be a big deal, but discrimination can lead to oppression, marginalization, and exclusion. Psychologist and author Dr. Tracey Gendron writes in her book *Ageism Unmasked: Exploring Age Bias and How to End It,* "Ageism against older people is widely prevalent, accepted, and based on a systemic value that idealizes youth over old age."[31]

Ageism is deeply embedded and flourishing in the minds and attitudes of each of us and is ubiquitous in our culture. We permit destructive attitudes about old age (e.g., aging is terrible and ugly) that we would never allow about race or sex. Author and activist Ashton Applewhite, in her book *This Chair Rocks: A Manifesto against Ageism,* points out that aging and disease do not go hand in hand. Aging itself is not a disease; otherwise, life would be a disease.[32] Even highly confined and constrained lives in older age can be rich and fulfilling.

People would live longer if older people in the United States were respected and revered, as in Japan. But ageism is about far more than longevity. It has damaging effects on health, exacerbating heart disease, diabetes, and Alzheimer's, as well as other illnesses. Gendron writes, "Ageism has severe and damaging consequences to our health and happiness throughout our entire lives."[33]

In our society, aging is seen as a bad thing. We see older people as unproductive, useless, and even pathetic. A colossal multibillion-dollar anti-aging industry has been created to combat aging. We have come to accept as normal that it's horrible to be old. We view old age as a period of decline, diminishment, and debility.

But we must embrace and celebrate getting older. Being ashamed, embarrassed, or anxious about getting old is as shortsighted as denying death. Aging can be a vibrant, purposeful, and joyful experience, full of new opportunities for growth, rich experiences, deep relationships, and meaningful contributions. We should feel proud of getting older and accumulating a variety of precious life experiences. It can be a time of engagement and creativity.

DECOUPLE AGING AND DEATH

We should not conflate aging and death. The psychologist and author James Hillman argues we must decouple dying from aging and restore the link between old age and depth of character.[34] Older people are depositories of stories and values. They have wisdom and experience that younger people lack. Older age involves decline and loss, but not uselessness. Older people who have lived rich and fulfilling lives of purpose and meaning have something to teach the young. They are role models of how to age well and be a nurturing and giving force in their families and communities.

How older people respond to the depletions of aging (loss of spouses and friends, reduced vision and hearing, loss of mobility, and so on) and the manner of their dying can give hope and fortitude to the young.[35] Older people can reveal to those who are younger that old age is not as bad as some people make it out to be and that death is something to face up to rather than turn away from in fear.

Above all, the old can teach the young to live fully up to the very end of life. Aging is not a disease. Dr. Tracey Gendron writes, "Aging is multidimensional and multidirectional."[36] Pioneering geriatrician Robert Butler wrote in 1975, "The tragedy of old age is not the fact that each of us must grow old and die, but that the process of doing so has been made unnecessarily and at times excruciatingly painful, humiliating, debilitating, and isolating."[37]

A PAINTER'S REMARKABLE STORY

In the winter of 1941, a seventy-one-year-old Frenchman was heading into a disastrous old age. After risky surgery that left him with severe abdominal pain, he was languishing in a wheelchair. German troops overran his beloved France, and, as the war years advanced, infections, pain, and anorexia ravaged his body. Old age left him disabled, decrepit, isolated, and uncertain about his future.

But something remarkable emerged from the fading older man in question. He was the French artist Henri Matisse. He recovered from being half dead and debilitated and went on in his seventies and eighties to revolutionize the art world. Matisse himself said the secret to his astonishing resurrection was aging itself. He thought that age brought him courage and enhanced his creativity.

The geriatrician Dr. Marc Agronin, from whom I learned the Matisse story, argues that aging brings strength.[38] He writes in his book *The End of Old Age*, "When we realize the truth of this message [that aging brings strength], we can begin to end the tired and constricted notions of 'old' that we internalize through our lifetime and that serve to denigrate and limit our aging self and perpetuate an ageist culture."[39]

"Aging brings strength." Think about that. It contradicts everything we've been taught by the media, advertising, and society's norms. Ageism teaches the precise opposite message: Aging brings weakness, frailty, uselessness, and decay. In reality, aging brings autonomy, agency, power, confidence, and freedom.

THE VILLAGE MOVEMENT

Another way to improve our chances of having a good death is to join "a village." In 1999, the first-ever "virtual retirement community," the Beacon Hill Village in Boston, began operating under the exciting notion that older people could help each other flourish while remaining in their own homes, not in an age-segregated community. Today, the rapidly growing Village-to-Village Network, founded to promote the Beacon Hill concept, has taken root in 270 US locations and has spread abroad as well. It is helping older people age in place and stay in their homes instead of moving into assisted living.

Joining a village (like the village I belong to, the Bethesda Metro Area Village in Bethesda, Maryland) is a way of gaining a "tribe," enriching your social life, and developing friendships. Many studies have shown that greater social relationships lead to a significant reduction in early death. The fast-growing village movement makes communities friendlier for older people who may not be as strong as they once were. Each village builds networks of support and provides volunteers to help older people get to a doctor's appointment, solve a computer headache, or change an out-of-reach light bulb.

There are many opportunities to gather for social occasions: potluck dinners, presentations by speakers, trips to museums and art galleries, lunches, book clubs, film groups, and other ways to help keep connected with others. Aging in place as long as possible helps us to live well, and, if we live well, we will more likely die well.

THE DEATH POSITIVE MOVEMENT

A new and constructive movement is underway to help people better prepare and plan for the end of their lives so they experience better deaths. This reform movement, led by patients, families, and even some pioneering doctors, aims to restore dignity and meaning to dying and to rid death of its awkwardness, shame, and dread.

One of the leaders of this movement is Caitlin Doughty, who wrote *Smoke Gets in Your Eyes* about the funeral industry. Doughty founded The Order of the Good Death to reframe what is possible at the end of life, and she cofounded the Death Positive Movement, which grew out of the Order and the surrounding community.

The tenets of the Death Positive Movement are as follows:[40]

1. Hiding death and dying behind closed doors does more harm than good to our society.

2. The culture of silence around death should be broken by discussion, gatherings, art, innovation, and scholarship.

3. Talking about and engaging with one's inevitable death is not morbid but displays a natural curiosity about the human condition.

4. The dead body is not dangerous, and people should be empowered (should they wish to be) to be involved in care for their own dead.

5. The laws that govern death, dying, and end-of-life care should ensure that a person's wishes are honored, regardless of sexual, gender, or racial or religious identity.

6. Deaths should be handled in a way that does not harm the environment.

7. Family and friends should know one's end-of-life wishes and have the necessary paperwork to back up those wishes.

8. Open, honest advocacy around death *can* make a difference and *can* change the culture.

These eight tenets of the Death Positive Movement are all excellent reasons why thinking about death and preparing and planning for it should not wait until the end of life.

DEATH CAFES AND "DEATH OVER DINNER"

Finding venues where people can discuss death openly without feeling awkward or weird is hard. Author Cory Taylor writes, "Despite the ubiquity of death, it seems strange that there are so few opportunities to publicly discuss dying."[41] Several initiatives have been started to deal with this problem. One of them is Death Cafes.[42]

Death Cafes provide community members, often strangers, of any background, religion, culture, or belief with the opportunity to meet in a safe and friendly environment to discuss thoughts and feelings about death and dying. The focus is on talking about death as a way to improve and enrich our daily lives. There is no agenda or objective. The topics are brought by any group member who may have something to share.

A Death Cafe can be a nonthreatening place to talk about how experiencing and witnessing death and dying feels. The goal is to increase awareness of death in order to help participants have more fulfilling lives. A Death Cafe is a discussion group rather than a grief support or counseling session, but participation can help you achieve a better death by simply talking about it honestly.

Another initiative, founded and led by author and death expert Michael Hebb, is Death over Dinner.[43] About seventy thousand people in thirty countries have participated in the Death Over Dinner movement since it began in 2013.[44] It aims to foster open and meaningful conversations about death and dying. It involves hosting intimate dinners where participants discuss end-of-life topics, allowing them to share their thoughts, fears, and wishes surrounding death. By breaking down the societal taboo around this subject, Death over Dinner provides a platform for individuals to connect, gain insights, and make informed decisions, ultimately promoting greater awareness and understanding of being mortal.

* * * * *

In this chapter, we have reasoned that, if you want a good death, you must live a good life, which requires planning and preparation. You can't leave it to chance. People tend to die the way they live. A good life is the foundation for a good death. To lead a good life, we should devote ourselves to building relationships, helping others, and working on meaningful projects and causes.

A key component of living and dying well is to be organized. We don't want to leave a big mess for our loved ones to clear up when we die. Decluttering, death cleaning, and getting organized are the topics of the next chapter.

CHAPTER 3

Decluttering, Death Cleaning, and Getting Organized

IT'S INCONSIDERATE TO LEAVE A HOUSE CLUTTERED WITH AN ENORmous collection of possessions to weed out. It's important not to burden loved ones with a big mess when death finally comes. This chapter is about getting our affairs in order by decluttering, death cleaning, and getting organized.

The term "death cleaning" was popularized by the book *The Gentle Art of Swedish Death Cleaning*, by Margareta Magnusson. She argues that we should have the foresight and generosity to eliminate most of our possessions before we die.

Far too many of us collect things at an alarming rate and in stunning quantities. Even worse, many people seem blind to the need to cull their stuff as they approach the end of their lives. Death cleaning and decluttering result in a home with a few items, all useful, meaningful, and valuable (e.g., they may carry strong emotional value).

Death cleaning is a gift to our survivors. If the term "death cleaning" is unappealing or even disagreeable, then call it decluttering, but, whatever the name, remember that every item we toss out is one less thing our survivors have to deal with.

Death cleaning means leaving our home decluttered and organized so that, after our death, our loved ones don't have to spend weeks or months burdened, angry, and irritated when their focus should be on how much they miss us and what we meant to them.

THE TOLL OF CLUTTER

Clutter has far more impact on people's lives than they generally realize. It makes us feel overwhelmed, stressed, and anxious. It damages our relationships, our health, and our enjoyment of life. How we organize the space around us affects our feelings and stress levels. Excess possessions prevent our homes from being places of comfort, joy, and relaxation. Clutter and confusion rob our attention and distract us from focusing on important things that matter to us, such as loved ones, friends, volunteering, projects, or whatever gives our life purpose and meaning.

Clutter steals our time because we research and buy things, and, once the items are in our home, we must maintain, clean, and organize them. The clutter keeps reminding us of open loops, uncompleted projects, and lost opportunities. This causes us to feel frustrated and unsatisfied.

Clutter happens because we think we may need the stuff at some later date, or it has some emotional value, or we paid good money for it (even though we might not have used it for years). We don't declutter because we don't have time; it's tedious and boring, and it's a low priority because we have more important things to do (or think we do).

As we age, we should stop buying things we don't need, never bring a new item into the house or apartment without throwing an item out, and get rid of obvious junk like old magazines or batteries. We should declutter and organize our stuff while we have the energy to do it.

REDUCING FAMILY DISCORD

A friend of mine got annoyed with her beloved and aging mother when her mother moved to an apartment and left her daughter to clear out the house. Her reaction was, "How could my mother impose on me months of tedious work that she should have done herself—time I simply don't have?"

Author and columnist Steven Petrow discovered how challenging clearing out a house can be. In his book *Stupid Things I Won't Do When I Get Old*, he describes how, after his parents died, he and his siblings were left with two houses packed to the rafters and a monumental job emptying them. They discovered that their parents not only had failed to declutter in their final years but also had added to their lifetime's worth of stuff.[1] It led Steven Petrow to become a devotee of death cleaning and decluttering.

Author and playwright Margaret Engel, who has researched and written on decluttering, says that daughters almost always get stuck with emptying houses when parents go into care homes or die. It's rare to see a son step up and handle this. There can be a lot of sibling resentment as daughters feel dumped on. Many services have emerged to declutter houses, from Clutter Busters to firms affiliated with real-estate companies that help people downsize from homes to condos or assisted-living facilities. The cost of these services, which can be about $4,000 per house, can be split among siblings so it's not automatically left to the daughters.

The brutal truth is that our survivors probably won't want our furniture, paintings, or fancy china. Instead, they will likely want small things that carry emotional value, such as select pieces of jewelry or some poignant letters. We need to identify what things we want certain family members to have and tell the whole family while we're alive so our children don't quarrel about them after we die. That is a nightmare we want to prevent.

We are responsible for doing everything we can to keep our loved ones from fighting over our estate after our death. Assigning objects in advance to family members will help to make conflicts less likely.

My friend Dave Nathan told me his deceased mother used to say, "I'm putting my house in dying condition." She meant that she was removing the junk in her house and making a list of who should get which furniture and other items. The upshot was that there was little to do after she died and no rancor among the three sons. His mother was considerate and gave a high priority to not burdening her sons. Nathan says, "Parceling out items in advance not only saves the arduous, time-consuming task of decluttering but also heads off later arguments, at a sensitive time, over who inherits what."[2]

Getting organized is an act of kindness and generosity to those we leave behind. It's harder to grieve fully if you are distracted by sibling hostility over who gets Grandma's jewelry or how to deal with Uncle Bertie's thousands of *National Geographic* magazines and vinyl records.

How selfless to die with our attic, garage, garden shed, basement, kitchen, study, bookshelves, and closets organized or cleared out.

BEING ORGANIZED

Being organized, neat, and tidy is only important as the means to an end, the "end" being a fulfilled and contented life. When we are organized, we can find what we need (our wallet, vacuum, grocery list) without frustration, stress, or wasting time. Organizational expert Maria Gracia says, "Eliminating clutter can be incredibly cathartic. Doing so puts you in control, brings better focus back to your life, and paves the way to more successes."[3]

The key to being organized is that everything we own should have a "home" in our house or apartment. This means that we know precisely where it is and can find it with little effort.

Gracia points out these five remarkable benefits that being organized has on our health and well-being:

1. *Being organized reduces our stress levels.* Removing clutter from our homes is like removing weights from our mind and body. Our stress levels decrease when we begin to get organized and continue to be organized. When stress levels decrease, so do our chances of other significant health challenges.

2. *Being organized helps us eat better.* Disorganized people are less likely to have planned for meals, shopped for healthy ingredients, or set aside time to cook, making them more likely to eat out or eat quick convenience foods that are not nutritionally sound.

3. *Being organized helps us be more active.* Organized people know how important it is to reach goals, including fitness goals that get them moving.

4. *Being organized helps us sleep better.* When we're organized, we launder our bed linens regularly, keep any clutter out of our bedroom, and have a relaxing evening routine that puts us in the right frame of mind to sleep.

5. *Being organized improves our relationships.* There is nothing more damaging to our emotional health than strained relationships. Having too much clutter can cause family tension.

How to Declutter

Organizing becomes much easier if we declutter first. The best option is to be both decluttered and organized so we have a calm, simple, and peaceful environment where everything has a home. The basic process is simple: Purge and organize. Some people start by trying to organize their belongings, but this is a mistake. Instead, start by purging—tossing out those things that, as author and tidying expert Marie Kondo puts it, no longer bring us joy. This can help to restore harmony, ease, and peacefulness to our lives.

The voluminous quantity of our possessions may be intimidating and lead to procrastination. Just looking at the amount of stuff needing to be sorted through can trigger intense feelings of being overwhelmed, leading to inaction. But death cleaning does not have to be accomplished all at once. It can be carried out over some years and a little bit at a time. Dividing the job into a series of small and manageable tasks makes sense. Perhaps we start with the garage, then tackle our clothes, followed by a significant thinning of our books, and so on. In this way, we will slowly but steadily death clean our home.

Minimalism

Decluttering ensures our survivors are not left with a terrible mess to clear up after we die. However, a minimalist approach to possessions is even better than decluttering. Minimalism isn't just about getting rid of clutter. It's about adding freedom and control to our lives. Author and minimalist Joshua Becker says that "minimalism" and "decluttering" are often used interchangeably, but there's a distinction. He says that decluttering focuses on removing possessions while minimalism helps us discover how little we actually need them.[4]

Minimalism is about regaining our energy, money, and time for things that really matter to us. It stands in stark contrast to its opposites: consumerism and materialism. Minimalism is becoming a popular lifestyle choice. Its essence isn't just less clutter but an internal journey to focus on what matters, how we spend our time, and how we relate to others. When done in the context of minimalism, decluttering means we will have more time to spend on what we love to do and who we want to be with.

Becker says that "minimalism is the intentional promotion of the things we most value and the removal of anything that distracts us from it." It requires a conscious decision because it's a lifestyle that militates against the overconsumption all around us. Becker writes, "Minimalism isn't about removing things you love. It's about removing the things that distract you from the things you love."[5]

A SIMPLIFICATION MINDSET

Getting rid of excess possessions is fundamentally about a mindset we need to develop as we grow older, a mindset that continually sifts through our activities to remove the things that don't matter and concentrate on what does. It's a mindset of intentional and deliberate simplification. Having a lot of possessions for most people is physically, financially, and emotionally draining. As we get older and less robust, simplifying our lives becomes increasingly essential.[6]

Decluttering and death cleaning are an important part of such life simplification, but a simplification mindset must extend to all aspects of our lives, including the size of our house or apartment, the size of our garden, our volunteer commitments, and the extent of our digital lives. Simplification helps to keep daily life manageable and less overwhelming.

PREPARING LEGAL DOCUMENTS

Once you are decluttered, it makes sense to get your legal will, your advance directive, and the appointment of your health-care agent completed while you still are in good health. It also makes sense to appoint your power of attorney for finances and name the beneficiaries on your retirement and bank accounts.

It's helpful to your surviving loved ones if you leave notes describing your vision for your memorial service, eulogy, and obituary, and leave a legacy letter and ethical will, plus notes on how you want to be treated when you are dying and how you want your body disposed of. When a loved one is dying, it's a time to say I love you, thank you, and other caring messages showing love. It isn't a time to be distracted, for example, by negotiations with a funeral director over how much he charges for burial or cremation.

Having a legal will and power of attorney and getting financial affairs in order are essential topics beyond this book's scope, but let me touch on them lightly. First, get help from a lawyer to do your legal will or use aids such as www.freewill.com. Remember that the legal requirements for a valid will may vary from state to state.

An astonishing 70 percent of people die without making a will (known as dying intestate), thus leaving their families, typically already roiling from the death, the added stress of dealing with the financial chaos and disarray that the death unleashes and possibly resulting in a distribution of estate assets that is different from what the deceased would want.[7]

A legal will describes how we want our money, assets, possessions, and property distributed after we die. In our will, we also identify who our executor—the person who will manage and implement our will—will be. We create wills to distribute our assets and reduce the possibility that our survivors may quarrel over who gets what. Thus, an important part of our legal will is to state who will get which items of our possessions or at least to offer guidance on resolving conflicts. Heirs may quarrel over items with emotional or economic value, and clear instructions can help settle such issues before relationships become damaged.

In their book, *A Beginner's Guide to the End*, BJ Miller and Shoshana Berger write, "There's no shortage of litigation between family members who feel slighted by a parent or spouse's decisions, or who harbor old resentments." They add, "Just because siblings are in their sixties doesn't mean that childhood wounds are healed."[8] Such wounds can lead to furious outbursts, smoldering anger, caustic conflicts, and even estrangement, all exacerbated by grief and sadness.

The bottom line is that you will need a competent lawyer to prepare a lucid, unambiguous, and effective legal will to reduce the risk of wasteful and exhausting litigation or estate mediation. Creating a legal will, like death cleaning and decluttering, is a gift to your loved ones that will likely save them needless suffering, time, and energy in settling your affairs.[9]

NECESSARY FILES

Getting organized means getting things like death cleaning, an advance directive, a legal will, an ethical will, and so on done and making sure the right people, including your doctors and loved ones, can access the information when needed. Keeping all your pertinent end-of-life paperwork in one place is another loving and thoughtful gift you can give your family to help them when you die.

Organizing guru Maria Gracia suggests the following checklist for organizing and managing your affairs so that loved ones know where to look for important papers and documents. You may not need all of the following information, or you may need more. Every family is different.

Personal Records

- Full legal name
- Social security number
- Legal residence
- Date and place of birth
- Names and addresses of spouse and children, and parents' names (specifically mother's maiden name)
- Assisted living facility/nursing home contact information/in-home care
- Birth and death certificates and certificates of marriage, divorce, citizenship, and adoption
- Care of pets (who and how)
- Durable power of attorney
- Employers and dates of employment
- Education and military records
- Funeral, burial, or cremation desires, with paperwork for each if you preplanned

- Guardianship of children (if they are not adults)
- A living will (advance directive) and other legal documents
- Passport
- Power of attorney documents
- Religious contacts (names and phone numbers)
- Medications taken regularly (be sure to update this regularly)
- Memberships in groups and awards received
- Names and phone numbers of close friends, relatives, doctors, lawyers, and financial advisors
- Obituary desires/wording/notes
- Organ donor information
- User names and passwords (banks, investments, social media accounts, etc.)
- Legacy letter (ethical will)
- Memorial service notes

Financial Records

- Banks and account numbers (checking, savings, credit union)
- Business or real estate owned
- Car title and registration
- Credit- and debit-card names and numbers
- Deed for home
- Income and assets (pension from employer, IRAs, 401(k)s, interest, etc.)
- Income tax returns (the last seven years)
- Insurance information (life, health, long-term care, home, car) with policy numbers and agents' names and phone numbers
- Investment income (stocks, bonds, property) and stockbrokers' names and phone numbers

- Medicare/Medicaid information
- Liabilities, including property tax—what is owed, to whom, and when payments are due
- Mortgages and debts—how and when they are paid
- Safe deposit box (location) and key
- Veteran's benefits
- Original legal will (it is much harder to probate a copy of a will if it can be done at all)
- Name of your accountant and lawyer

You should keep all your files in a safe place your loved ones are familiar with so they know where to find all the information they need as you age and require help.

My friend and author Diane MacEachern created a "red folder" with everything her children must handle when she dies. It has given her peace of mind to know that, if she dies unexpectedly, her children won't have to track down everything they would need to deal with the business side of her death.

The red folder includes her legal will, her advance directive, the name and contact information for her lawyer, the name and contact information for her accountant and bookkeeper, and her financial planner's name and phone number. It also includes the following:

- A list of the names and email addresses of everyone who should be contacted to let them know she has died
- A list of all her social media accounts and passwords
- A list of her bank accounts and credit cards
- A list of her passwords for each of her financial accounts and other important online sites
- A list of anything she has financed and information on her car lease
- A list of her insurance policies, agents, and contact information

- A list of a couple of real-estate agents to help her children sell the house
- A list of the contractors who know the house (plumber, painter, carpenter, landscaper) to do any necessary repairs
- Account information for utilities and other ongoing service providers
- A list of the many benefits of the house (location, near public transportation, energy efficiency, native plants garden, current maintenance, size, etc.), mostly for marketing purposes
- A list of where to donate furniture, books, etc., with the names and contact information of services that can help (charities, pick-up services, book drop-offs, etc.)
- A list of items they might not realize are valuable or have family value and shouldn't donate
- A list of items she would like to go to other family members if her children don't want them, specifying the family member to give them to
- Some cash to cover immediate incidental expenses

MacEachern has also included some suggestions for a memorial service, including musical selections and readings, whom to invite, and possible locations. She has made some suggestions regarding the disposition of her body. And she has made sure that a loved one or trusted friend knows how her house works (how to open and lock it, how to turn the water off and on, how to turn the heat on and off, etc.).

Bureaucracy after Death

Even if you're organized, the logistics and paperwork can be overwhelming, which is not a good experience when you are also knocked sideways with grief. Journalist and playwright Allison Engel reports in *The Washington Post* that, after her husband died, despite having all her affairs in good order, she experienced an absurd amount of red tape.[10] She writes that she had to deal "with ridiculous tech barriers and nonsensical policies that make the days, weeks and months after [the death of a loved one] a marathon of frustrating phone calls."

Engel says, "We thought our financial affairs were organized and well documented, but we've endured months of painful and frustrating experiences with banks, insurance companies, employers, and the Social Security Administration." She warns that, at some point, we'll all have to handle "the oppressive red tape when a loved one or friend dies."

Engel recommends the following:

1. Keep an updated list of recurring credit-card charges organized by each card.

2. Make sure the surviving spouse or partner has a credit card she applied for in her own name.

3. Get a password manager to hold all your user names and passwords, and ensure your survivors have the master password.

4. Purchase at least five or six copies of the death certificate. Although, lately, some companies will allow you to email scanned copies, most require you to send an actual certificate bearing an embossed seal or inked signature.

5. Ensure you have birth and marriage certificates, adoption or divorce documents, and Social Security cards. These documents may have gotten lost after many decades of marriage and multiple moves. It can take weeks to get copies from the various agencies. So, do an inventory now and make sure you have them all.

6. Don't put these important documents, or a will, in a safety-deposit box. For survivors, getting access to a safety-deposit box can be a lengthy process, particularly if your loved one misplaced the key.

7. Medicare will continue to send bills and notices to the deceased's last address, so continue to pay for the US Postal Service to forward mail even after you (the partner, child, or next-of-kin handling the red tape) have moved from that address. Even if you've informed Social Security of an address change (and Social Security

is supposed to coordinate with Medicare on your address), the mail from Medicare does not update.

Decluttering, death cleaning, and getting organized help our loved ones and remove a significant burden from them, for which they will be grateful. The more we can death clean, be organized, and practice minimalism and simplicity, the easier it is for our loved ones to grieve freely and fully without being overwhelmed with all that must be done when we die. When thinking about the end of our lives, we must consider how it impacts those we love. To do so is to act with grace, honor, and thoughtfulness.

* * * * *

Being organized and decluttered will help us achieve a good death. Another component of achieving a good death is to have "the conversation" about death and dying with our loved ones and doctors and complete an advance directive. We turn to these topics next.

CHAPTER 4

Advance Directives, "The Conversation," and Health-Care Agents

AN ADVANCE DIRECTIVE IS A LEGALLY VALID FORM THAT ALLOWS patients to choose the type of medical care they wish to receive at the end of life when they can no longer speak for themselves. You may be wondering why advance directives appear so early in the book, especially when you may recall from the Preface that I've organized this book on the continuum from life to death.

Advance directives appear here because they should be completed when we are young. Life is fragile, and we never know when unexpected events might happen. It may seem unnecessary for young people to complete advance directives, but the most famous cases in US legal history concerning end-of-life care involve three young women: Karen Ann Quinlan, Nancy Cruzan, and Terri Schiavo.

They would be far less well-known today in legal circles if they had completed advance directives. So much of the energy and spirit behind the lawsuits they and their families got enmeshed in would have been absent had the three women made it clear before ending up in hospital how they wanted to be treated on their deathbeds. Advance directives may not have been available to Quinlan and Cruzan (after all, their experiences led to the development of advance-directive law), but Schiavo could have completed one. This chapter discusses the importance of talking with your loved ones and doctors about your wishes and aspirations for the end of life and how you want to be treated.

FEW AMERICANS HAVE COMPLETED ADVANCE DIRECTIVES

Karen Ann Quinlan, Nancy Cruzan, and Terri Schiavo were all in their twenties when they had personal disasters and were incapacitated and comatose. Karen Quinlan became vegetative in 1975 and was kept alive for ten years. Nancy Cruzan became vegetative in 1983 and was kept alive for eight years. Terri Schiavo became vegetative in 1990 and was kept alive for fifteen years. The lack of an advance directive in each case resulted in the courts stepping in to decide their fate. All three cases led to an upsurge in the use of advance directives, yet two out of three US adults have not completed an advance directive. Given the stakes, this is a shockingly low number.

Americans are fascinated by death and dying—as we can see from the TV news and films that emphasize fatal accidents and murders—yet conversations about death and dying and what people want at the end of life typically are rare. Clinical psychologist and friend Patricia Steckler, PhD, says, "It's so interesting to me that people who've been proactive in life choices become utterly obsequious with a 'whatever happens, happens' attitude at the end of life. It's as if exercising some choice or making plans is not an option."[1]

WHY ARE WE SO TONGUE-TIED?

While our attention is drawn to death and dying, talking about achieving a good death is taboo. Why are we so reticent and tongue-tied? There are several reasons. First, parents don't want to cause their kids anxiety and discomfort. Second, children are reluctant to raise such an intimate topic with their parents for fear of somehow tempting the gods to bring it about. Third, doctors are taciturn on the subject because death signifies that they have failed to save their patient, and no one likes to admit failure. But this lack of conversation leads to negative outcomes for everyone.

The difference between a hard death and a good death often depends on whether patients have talked with loved ones about what they want at the end of life. We should not be discussing a sick or injured person's end-of-life wishes for the first time when they're in an ICU. That's too late.

We must live so as to be ready for death at any time. On April 14, 1912, William John Rogers sent some friends a postcard from the *Titanic*. "Dear Friends," Rogers wrote, "Just a line to show that I'm alive & kicking and going grand." Tragically, the next day, the *Titanic* sank, and Rogers drowned. This story underscores a profound truth about life. One day we can be doing well; the next, we can die.

ADVANCE CARE PLANNING

Patient-directed care (agency over our health care) is essential and requires that we have the tools and information to choose our end-of-life journey according to our priorities and values. That includes understanding the importance of advance directives as well as their weaknesses. Advance care planning includes completing an advance directive, deciding the treatments we would want or not want, deciding on a health-care agent, and sharing our values and preferences with loved ones and doctors.

Former Maryland state legislator, author, and emergency-medicine physician Dan Morhaim writes, "We should be encouraging and assisting our patients to complete an advance directive and to make sure these forms are electronically securely stored and readily available across the healthcare continuum 24/7."[2] Advance care planning is the key to reducing pain and suffering at the end of life. As Morhaim says, there would be less need for palliative sedation or other similar measures discussed in chapter 8 if people would complete advance directives while they have the mental capacity to do so.[3]

Advance care planning involves making decisions about the health care you want to receive at the end of life or in a medical crisis. When people are diagnosed with a serious illness, they should prioritize early advance care planning conversations with their family and doctors. Studies have shown that patients participating in advance care planning are more likely to receive care aligned with their wishes.[4]

As noted, an advance directive is a legally valid form that allows patients to choose the type of medical care they wish to receive at the end of life when they can no longer speak for themselves. It has three parts: selecting a health-care agent or proxy, deciding on the care wanted at the end of life, and choosing what happens to the body after death.

We know life is unpredictable, yet many of us have not prepared advance directives.[5] The shortsighted reason for this lack of preparation is obvious. Not doing our advance directives and other end-of-life planning makes it easier for us to deny that we will die.[6]

The consequences of not creating an advance directive include increasing the probability that we will die in a hospital ICU hooked up to tubes and ventilators, unable to speak, and alone. Completing an advance directive helps to avoid a dehumanizing and painful death. At the end of life, not having an advance directive and not having had "the conversation" can lead to overly aggressive medical interventions that might do more harm than good. And no advance directive means that our loved ones are left struggling alone, wondering what we would have wanted.[7] They will yearn for our guidance when we are near death and when they have to make difficult decisions on our behalf about how our life should end. It's worth filling out an advance directive if only as a loving gift to those we cherish.

EXPRESSING OUR GOALS FOR LIVING

Advance care planning allows us to articulate our goals in life, and these goals then drive the plan of care to determine what treatments can achieve those goals. Palliative care doctor Shahid Aziz writes, "Goals of care drive the plan of care."[8] Often, advance directives involve a checklist where we indicate, for example, that we don't want our life extended if we are in a persistent vegetative state. But this is of limited value.

An advance directive should include our *goals for living* to clarify what is meaningful to us. For example, concerns often revolve around being able to communicate easily with loved ones, the ability to toilet and bathe, incontinence of both urine and stool, the ability to enjoy food, and mobility. What level of physical functioning is acceptable to us with life-prolonging interventions? Perhaps being bedridden and having to use a bedpan is acceptable, but anything worse than that (e.g., being bed-ridden and needing diapers) is not. What about mental functioning? Perhaps being able to recognize loved ones but unable to communicate with them is acceptable, but being unable to recognize them is unacceptable.

DNR Litmus Test

Dr. Eleanor Tanno, a doctor and educator specializing in helping people complete their advance directives, says there's one statement we should be able to express in our advance directive, and that is, "I would want to live as long as I could still . . . (then complete the sentence with what is most important to you)."[9] Tanno says this is one of the most critical statements to define our end-of-life wishes. She has termed it our "Do Not Resuscitate (DNR) Litmus Test."

Our loved ones and doctors must understand our personal values and goals—our goals of care. If we say to our family, "In the event of a terminal illness, I do not want heroic measures," it's hard to know precisely what we mean. Tanno advises that we focus on conveying our values and goals instead of discussing "heroic measures" or other medical treatments. One way to name those concretely is to create the DNR Litmus Test.

The DNR Litmus Test identifies which basic activities represent an acceptable quality of life. Our health-care agent can subject our likely medical outcomes to that test. For example, your life would be worth living as long as you could still (pick some functions, such as the following):

- Recognize your spouse, grandchildren, and other family members and friends
- Talk to your family and friends
- Take yourself to the bathroom (i.e., not be incontinent)
- Get out of bed
- Walk
- Swallow
- Feed yourself
- Taste food
- Use a cell phone
- Read books
- Live on your own (i.e., not in a nursing home)

To show how the DNR Litmus Test is applied, consider how a doctor's proposal could "fail" the Litmus Test. Suppose the doctor offers a medical treatment unlikely to restore your function level to pass the Litmus Test. In that case, your medical decision-maker can decline that treatment with a clear conscience. Say your Litmus Test included something physical, such as the ability to garden. If the doctor offers invasive surgery to treat a heart problem, but you have already suffered a severe stroke that has rendered you immobile, then your decision-maker can decline the surgery as it did not pass the Litmus Test.

The DNR Litmus Test helps uncover what is critical to your quality of life, including physical, cognitive, and relationship activities. Discussing your DNR Litmus Test with your health-care agent is essential, so it can be applied to your medical care if you cannot talk for yourself.

EMPOWERMENT THROUGH ADVANCE DIRECTIVES

Author and emergency-medicine doctor Dan Morhaim says, "Our culture celebrates personal freedom and autonomy. Yet, in this one area [death and dying], we collectively abdicate those values. Only about 40 percent of Americans overall—and about 20 percent in communities of color—take advantage of advance directives for empowerment, control, and respect for individual values."[10]

If you want to fill out an advance directive but are unsure where to start, the following websites can be helpful: The Conversation Project (theconversationproject.org—more on this later in the chapter), AARP (aarp.org), Compassion & Choices (candc.org), and MyDirectives.com. You can add your own personal touches to your advance directive. For example, Morhaim added, "I want to be taken outdoors as much as possible, and if that can't be done, put me where I can see outside. I want vodka and medical cannabis. I want control of the remote and a bite of chocolate every day. I have a list of music I'd like to hear and a list of people I'd like to see—and maybe a few I can do without."[11]

ADDING A DEMENTIA PROVISION[12]

A person with Alzheimer's or another dementia faces the terrifying prospect of becoming a dysfunctional and different person. Advanced dementia can bring hellish consequences to patients and loved ones alike. People suffering from dementia have their personalities, characters, and memories eviscerated. This impacts not only the brain but also the entire nervous system. Some may rage at their loved ones (after a lifetime of being gentle and affectionate), while others may be reduced to childlike dependence (after a lifetime of being self-confident and strong).

The Alzheimer's Association says that Alzheimer's cannot be cured and that one in three seniors dies with (and many from) Alzheimer's or another form of dementia.[13] The organization also notes that improving health through exercise and nutritious eating can lower the risk of dementia.

Patients with dementia are as likely as any other patient to be given harsh medical treatments in which doctors assume that the goal of care is to prolong the *quantity* of life by as much as possible. Shockingly, nine out of every ten patients with dementia have at least one medical procedure in the last week of their lives, like hip or knee replacement, cardiac pacemaker implantation, mechanical ventilation, or insertion of feeding tubes.[14]

Advanced medical technology can now extend the lives of patients with dementia almost indefinitely, but this is both hideous and irrational. It is hard to imagine patients seeing themselves in the future suffering from end-stage dementia and wanting a life-prolonging and painful treatment. Most of us would shake our heads in horror and say, "No thanks, just let me die peacefully, swiftly, and naturally." Doctors should not automatically assume that all people with advanced dementia want their lives extended as much as possible and want to receive aggressive medical treatments to keep them alive, with no thought given to their quality of life.

If patients with advanced dementia documented their wishes earlier in their lives (when they still had decision-making capability) for a gentle, dignified, and peaceful death, that should be respected. Such documentation would be in the form of a dementia provision added to the advance directive. One of the best such provisions comes from Compassion & Choices and can be found on their website.[15]

With such provisions, patients can articulate in writing their wishes for treatment, feeding, ventilation, antibiotics, and other interventions should they later suffer from advanced dementia. All people have the right to say they are unwilling to experience significantly reduced mental and emotional function—and eventually become a different person—because of Alzheimer's or other dementia.

DECIDING ON THE "LINE" AND FINDING A PEACEFUL EXIT PLAN

Some people with advanced dementia would rather be dead than suffer through the end stages of their disease—being unable to walk, incapable of feeding themselves, unable to recognize loved ones, and with their mental and emotional faculties largely destroyed and suffering from fecal incontinence and significant personality and behavior changes. Life-prolonging treatments under these circumstances are neither rational nor wise. If a patient has advanced dementia, the best approach is to let the person die naturally and not do anything to impede that from happening while providing as much comfort as possible.

Patients with dementia usually suffer a glacially slow decline. Patients will draw the line differently, marking the start of a status that is no longer acceptable to them and where they no longer want to receive life-prolonging interventions. It's crucial to document in your dementia provision (part of your advance directive) where you want to draw the line so that your caregivers, health-care agent, and medical providers know what you want.[16]

We need to help people determine—in advance of the loss of decision-making capacity due to dementia—the point at which they would like to forgo treatments and allow a natural death. Both patients and doctors must understand the importance of documenting this preference before mental capacity is lost.

The way to achieve a peaceful and dignified death with Alzheimer's and other dementia is to articulate in writing and conversations with loved ones the "line" past which you do not wish to live. This must be done while the disease is still in its early stages.

Enforcing an Advance Directive and Dementia Provision

The dementia provision must be executed when the patient is fully competent and must be advocated for by the patient's family to ensure it is honored. Doctors should embrace the legal end-of-life wishes of their patients with dementia who have proclaimed their desire to forgo treatments or voluntarily stop eating and drinking (for those still capable).

Patients can refuse treatment, even if it might save their life. If you don't want specific medical interventions and say so in your advance directive, doctors should not give them to you. Kathryn Tucker, an Oregon attorney specializing in advocacy for terminally ill people, urges that any advance directive and its dementia provision make clear that the instructions are to be followed. If they are ignored or thwarted, the survivors should take legal action to hold accountable anybody who prevented the implementation of the patient's wishes in tort and professional disciplinary actions.[17] Legal action against the medical provider may result in punitive payouts.

Wrongful-Prolongation-of-Life Lawsuits

As death expert and patient advocate Althea Halchuck writes, "Sometimes, resuscitating someone only prolongs a much-wanted death. The law is becoming clearer: The hospital's and doctor's responsibility is to check your advance directive and follow your wishes—or suffer the consequences."[18] Wrongful-prolongation-of-life lawsuits are increasing. Halchuck says medical-care providers should take note and beware. Advance directives give competent adult patients the right to accept or reject medical treatment and to choose a surrogate to speak for them when they become incapacitated.

This right was codified in 1990 when Congress passed the Patient Self-Determination Act, encouraging the creation of advance directives before a person becomes incapacitated and unable to make medical care and end-of-life preferences known.[19]

Medical providers must follow a legally executed advance directive or medical order, such as a do-not-resuscitate (DNR) order. Doctors cannot override a patient's wishes, later claiming they were acting in good faith. Faye Girsh, an activist for the right to a peaceful death and founder of the

Hemlock Society of San Diego, says, "The Catholic Church continues to wield enormous power and is taking over community hospitals where even advance directives are not honored."[20] But, as already noted, there are legal and financial risks to doctors and hospitals for not obtaining, not reviewing, and not following patients' advance directives.[21]

SELECTING A HEALTH-CARE AGENT

A crucial part of an advance directive is selecting who will be your health-care agent. Also called a health proxy, medical advocate, surrogate, or medical power of attorney, your health-care agent is the person you appoint to speak for you if you cannot make medical decisions because you are too ill or are unconscious or lack capacity to make decisions. Your health-care agent should know you well, know your values, and be able to carry out the wishes expressed in your advance directive. If you don't appoint a health-care agent, then there is a chance you will receive treatments to prolong your life rather than allow a natural death.

You want someone comfortable with the responsibility of representing you and able to make tough decisions on your behalf. Choose someone to be your health-care agent who is assertive when talking with doctors, even if the doctors are authoritarian and overbearing.

If you have no health-care agent, many states provide a ranking of which of your closest relatives have priority to make health-care decisions on your behalf. If no family member is willing to come forward and make a decision, doctors will default to doing everything they can with all the pain and suffering that goes with it.

Another skill your health-care agent will need is the strength to stand up to others who may try to intimidate them, such as an estranged or emotionally detached sibling who flies in from far away and disagrees with what is in your advance directive. (I discuss these so-called "seagull" relatives more in chapter 6.) Doctors are familiar with this troubling experience. After spending years neglecting the dying person, a relative suddenly appears in the ICU and wants to take over, ordering the doctors to "do everything possible" to save the patient, even though that isn't what the patient wants. Your health-care agent must have the backbone and fortitude to deal with this kind of unwelcome challenge.

It is not okay when family members insist on aggressive treatments for patients who are actively dying and have made it clear in their advance directive that they don't want to be overmedicalized near the end of their lives. A vital responsibility of a health-care agent is to make sure patients who are weak and in declining health are protected from harsh, aggressive, futile treatments.

Your closest relatives may not always be the best health-care agents. They may not be competent to represent you assertively and accurately. They may be too timid to stand up to doctors who recommend a treatment inconsistent with your advance directive. There can also be questionable financial motives, like a daughter facing a possible decade of expensive payments to a memory-care facility for her father, or a son who will continue to benefit financially from his mother's Social Security checks. Health-care agents should be guided by the wishes of the dying and not by any selfish motives.

THE LIMITS OF ADVANCE DIRECTIVES

Advance directives aren't a complete solution because sometimes they get ignored, and sometimes patients change their minds.[22] But even if they are not working as well as we would like, completing an advance directive is helpful because it can stimulate and encourage family members to think and hopefully talk about how patients want their lives to end. The essential part of advance care planning is not completing an advance directive and checking boxes but the conversation, stimulated by filling out an advance directive, between patients and their health-care agents, their loved ones, and their doctors about the patient's goals and values.

These conversations allow patients to describe in general terms what states of health are unacceptable and what functional capacities they want to have to make staying alive worth it. As discussed earlier, they may prefer to die peacefully and gently if they don't have these functional capabilities. Advance directives are often vague concerning the steps between being healthy and being dead. They tend only to cover issues that arise if we are close to death. They deal with extreme circumstances, such as what to do if a loved one has a terminal illness or is in a persistent vegetative state, but what about all the steps before that?

Your health-care agent and doctors can only learn so much from your advance directive. It has to be supplemented with conversations. Advance directives alone cannot guarantee that end-of-life wishes will be respected. Even a highly detailed advance directive will never cover all the medical situations patients might find themselves in, so having an ongoing conversation with a health-care agent, loved ones, and doctors is essential. Such discussions will better prepare all of those people to make wise decisions on your behalf when you can no longer speak for yourself.

ICU physician Dr. Jessica Zitter points out another weakness of advance directives for patients in nursing homes. Nursing homes highlight advance-directive completion rates with great pride because they think this metric shows how much they pay attention to the needs of their patients. However, Zitter points out that those advance directives from nursing homes all have a "cookie-cutter similarity." Almost all of them, she writes, indicate that the patient wants everything possible done to prolong life. Rarely is a treatment, such as CPR, considered unacceptable, regardless of the patient's prognosis. Nursing homes are paid to care for patients as long as they remain alive, so they have a perverse financial incentive to encourage their patients to ask that "everything be done."[23]

"THE CONVERSATION"

An advance directive is a tool to help us convey to our family and medical providers how we want to be cared for and treated at the end of life. It is a starting point for ongoing dialogue and conversation with our doctors and loved ones. Our goals and priorities may change as we get older. For example, a treatment deemed unacceptable, such as being intubated, may, over time, not seem so bad. An ongoing conversation with loved ones can reveal these shifting priorities so that our caregivers can know our current wishes.

Patients who discuss their preferences with their doctors and loved ones will likely suffer less in their last weeks and days of life than those who do not.[24] In his book *Being Mortal*, surgeon Dr. Atul Gawande writes, "People who had substantive discussions with their doctor about their end-of-life preferences were far more likely to die at peace and in control of their situation and to spare their family anguish."[25]

The Baby Boom generation is living longer (a good thing), but caring for them will become more expensive. In the United States, about one-third of the Medicare budget (now approaching a stunning one trillion dollars) is spent in the last six months of life.[26] This spending can be significantly reduced by rejecting unnecessary surgeries, tests, and treatments. These substantial financial savings would allow the nation to spend more on essential health goals like cancer research and fighting childhood diseases. However, such savings can only happen if patients have articulated their end-of-life goals and minimum acceptable levels of physical, mental, and emotional function with their loved ones and doctors.[27]

Hospice and palliative care doctor Shahid Aziz says early conversations about the end of life "can prevent crisis-driven, desperate, irrational, emotional, and expensive decision-making."[28] According to *The Lancet*, about 10 percent of annual health expenditures in higher-income countries is spent on the less than 1 percent who die. Many patients have surgery, radiation, chemo, and other interventions up to the end, meaning a good death becomes impossible. Palliative care helps but is not used widely enough.[29]

Medicare pays doctors a modest fee to discuss advanced illness and end-of-life preferences with patients. Even though there are no quality metrics to measure how doctors perform at this task, the fee should be higher and more in line with the compensation physicians receive for doing tests and treatments.[30]

Discussing our values and priorities related to illness, frailty, and dying is essential while we are comparatively young and healthy. The more your family hears you speak about it, the more likely you will get what you want.

The longer the conversation about end-of-life wishes is delayed, the more challenging such conversations become. However, even scraps and fragments of ideas can help your health-care agent do the right thing. To say things like, "Do everything you can to keep me alive as long as possible," or "I never want to be on a mechanical ventilator," or "Keep me free of pain even if the morphine hastens my death" can help your health-care agent make the decisions you want and markedly reduce the decision-making burden on them. In these conversations, patients share their vision of the death they want with their doctors and family. Hopefully, that vision will include potential exit strategies, such as, "When I'm close to death, don't give me antibiotics if I get pneumonia." I'll say more about exit strategies at the end of this chapter.

Gawande wryly writes, "If end-of-life discussions were an experimental drug, the FDA would approve it."[31] Such conversations, if held regularly, can help the family form a vision of how their loved one wants to die so that the health-care agent can be in a position to push hard on medical providers to give the patient the end of life that the patient desires. In her book *That Good Night*, hospice physician Sunita Puri describes how she fought to overcome her reluctance to talk to her parents about how they wanted to be treated at the end of their lives and how having this conversation with them brought her "a deep peace."[32]

STARTING THE CONVERSATION

People don't have the conversation because they fear death. They deal with this dread by avoiding any discussion of death and dying. But one easy way to start the conversation is to discuss advance directives. For example, if your heart stops, do you want CPR? Do you want to be on a ventilator?

Conversations about death and dying must become routine if we want to achieve our goal of making it easier for people to attain peaceful and good deaths. A good resource in this area is an ambitious program called The Conversation Project, founded by the Pulitzer Prize–winning *Boston Globe* columnist Ellen Goodman. It encourages people to talk openly with their loved ones and doctors about how they want to be treated at the end of life. The Conversation Project recommends that the end-of-life conversation begin when a person is in good health and suggests the following ways to start it:[33]

1. I need your help with something.

2. Remember how Aunt Paula died? Do you think it was a good death or a hard death? How would you like yours to be different?

3. I was thinking about what happened to Grandpa, which made me realize . . .

4. I need to think about the future. Will you help me?

Author and activist Diane MacEachern points out that the nature of the conversation will depend on the people having it. How easy is it for the dying person to talk about death? How easy is it for the other person? And it is not one conversation, but many over time. When you're not sick, the conversation seems a little abstract and focused on the future. That's a very different scenario from the conversation we would have if we had a fatal disease or had been in an accident that left us with only days to live. Also, conversations with relatives in their twenties differ from those with them when they are more mature.

Who is responsible for getting these death-and-dying conversations started? Medicare requires primary-care physicians to ask about end-of-life care decisions during annual wellness visits. But the responsibility can't be dumped on family doctors. All doctors who work with chronically ill patients should be talking about the end of life. And family members must talk with each other.

DOCTORS AND MORTALITY

It's challenging to achieve a good death if we don't know we are dying, and doctors are reluctant to tell a patient that he is dying and nothing more can be done. Aggravating this situation is the fact that doctors consistently overestimate how long their patients will survive and how well they will recover function.[34] Studies show that most doctors are overly optimistic when making end-of-life prognoses—meaning their patients' lives are shorter than predicted. A prognosis predicts the likely course of an illness, and doctors typically cannot prognosticate with much certainty or accuracy.[35] Overestimating how long a person has to live might kindle overtreatment and delay the consideration of hospice care.[36]

Palliative care doctor BJ Miller says that there's no evidence that a doctor being honest about a terminal condition destroys a patient's hope, "and plenty to suggest that it can bring patient and doctor closer."[37] Candidly and sympathetically discussing bad news is the right way for doctors to talk with their patients unless a patient has explicitly requested not to be informed. Some patients may not want to know their prognosis or even details of their treatment, but most patients *will* want their doctors to tell them everything, including prognosis, recommended treatment, alternative treatments, the consequences and benefits of no treatment, and the quality of life and life expectancy under each scenario.

Doctors should provide patients nearing the end of their lives with honest and appropriate information about their diseases. This allows patients to address the final part of their lives and get their affairs in order. As author and hospice nurse Barbara Karnes says, "We are doing our patients a disservice by not telling them medicine has given them all it has to offer." Doctors are scared of death themselves, fear legal repercussions from ornery and conflicting family members, and worry that their prognoses might be wrong. Occasionally, they can be paternalistic, thinking they know better than patients what's good for them.

Doctors are taught little about mortality and death in medical school. Dr. Gawande begins *Being Mortal* with the words, "I learned about a lot of things in medical school, but mortality wasn't one of them. . . . Our textbooks had almost nothing on aging or frailty or dying."[38] Author and geriatrician Dr. Louise Aronson makes a similar point. She writes in *Elderhood*, "Ironically, despite the medicalization of dying, most doctors have little training in death."[39]

Not only doctors but also a patient's friends and family must grasp that it's morally wrong to hide information from patients for fear of upsetting them and to risk delaying or impeding the creation of end-of-life options. Patients cannot make sound health decisions without being informed. Palliative care doctor Ira Byock notes that doctors have "an aversion to talking about dying and death." Medical schools could change that reluctance by giving their students more training in palliative care. Doctors need to know if patients want to die gently and how to provide that option. Byock writes in his book *The Best Care Possible*:

> Most medical schools do not require hospice or palliative care rotations, many do not even offer them as electives. Medical schools generally

provide a lecture or two on pain management and discuss the ethics of end-of-life decisions and palliative and end-of-life topics within other courses. The total course content of these topics probably amounts to fifteen to twenty-five hours over the four years of medical school curriculum.[40]

Byock wrote that in 2012 and things have improved since then, but not nearly enough. Medical schools must teach doctors to have these conversations and not fear them. The ICU physician Jessica Zitter says she sees many cases where patients' bodies are being kept alive by breathing machines, feeding tubes, dialysis, and antibiotics "despite poor prognoses for recovery or return to their previous function."[41] But, she adds poignantly, "I so often wish that these patients had given some indication to a loved one or a doctor of how they would feel about being kept alive in this condition. Surveys show that almost no one wants that, and yet without a clear opt-out, we doctors feel obligated to keep such patients alive."

WAYS TO SUPPLEMENT AN ADVANCE DIRECTIVE

An advance directive gives a rough sense of how we want to be treated in a few medical circumstances. Still, it's not a doctor's order, and it's unavoidably hazy in many situations we might find ourselves in. As we become sicker and closer to death, we should supplement our advance directive with other tools, such as a DNR order and a physician order for life-sustaining treatment (POLST). Doctors sign both of these, so they carry considerable authority and, thus, are likely to be honored by hospitals and other medical-care providers.

A MOLST is a medical order for life-sustaining treatment and is identical to a POLST. A MOLST and a POLST refer to a doctor's medical treatment orders to be allowed or prohibited. For a patient who has an incurable disease, who is in frail health, or who is within a year or two of dying, having a POLST or MOLST is vital. The POLST or MOLST is usually (depending on the state) a one-page, double-sided, bright pink form that describes a patient's preferences regarding treatments like ventilators, CPR, and feeding tubes. Emergency medical technicians, paramedics, and other first responders are legally required to do everything they can to keep a person alive unless there is a signed doctor's order saying not to. POLST.org provides state-specific POLST and MOLST forms that are, as already noted, signed by doctors.

A "Do Not Resuscitate Order" or DNR (also called Allow Natural Death or AND) directs your medical-care team not to give you CPR (cardiopulmonary resuscitation) if your heart stops beating. If you don't want your chest aggressively compressed (and your ribs likely broken), your heart electrically shocked, and tubes inserted down your throat to keep you breathing, then you need a DNR. A doctor signs a DNR order when CPR is not in accordance with the patient's wishes, but it's only good for a particular admission at a particular time. If patients want to retain a DNR order, regardless of the facility or institution they're in, it's wise to ask the doctor to fill out a POLST or MOLST. Choosing "full code" as opposed to "no code" (or DNR) means that you want to be kept alive regardless of the cost in pain or suffering.

WHERE TO PUT YOUR PAPERWORK

It takes effort to complete an advance directive, a dementia provision, a POLST/MOLST form, and a DNR. All that effort will be wasted if no one can find the documents. So give all your completed forms, along with any letters similar to those in Appendices I and II, to your loved ones, health-care agent, and doctors. Ask your doctors to upload all these documents, including your advance directive, into their electronic medical system so that they become part of your chart and can be easily accessed by a new doctor you might be seeing. Registering your completed forms online with the US Living Will Registry or MyDirectives.com is also wise, as it allows them to be accessed from anywhere.

The late death and dying activist Rosalind Kipping advised, "Make many copies of your POLST and carry one on your person at all times. I have one in my wallet and in a side pocket of my purse with a label on it that says POLST. My wallet also has a POLST label where I have my driver's license. I am very serious about first responders finding it. I also have one on my refrigerator and in the auto front compartment. So, in case of an accident, it will be found by first responders. Give copies to your children and to other doctors."[42]

Your advance directive should be updated regularly, especially when health, values, and relationships change. MyDirectives.com sends a reminder every year or two, and you can change your advance directive anytime by logging on, which is easy to do.

Organ Donation[43]

Donating your organs to a person in need is generous, kind, and honorable because it saves lives, but, for this to be possible, you have to be in a hospital when you die. Patients who die at home, says palliative care doctor BJ Miller, "are not within range of equipment that keeps the organs viable and safe for the intended recipient."[44]

Your loved ones may not realize that your body in the hospital may be quickly taken away after you die so your organs can be successfully harvested. If family or friends want to spend some quiet, reflective, quality time with your body immediately after your death or anoint your body with sweet-smelling oils, as suggested in chapter 9, they may find it's not possible.

Exit Strategy

Author and hospice doctor Samuel Harrington argues in his book, *At Peace: Choosing a Good Death after a Long Life*, that we should each consider an exit strategy. By that, he means an illness for which we will decline treatment. When aggressive medical treatment like surgery results in complications and inadequate benefits, we should consider passive care, then hospice care, and then an exit opportunity.[45] We each need to visualize an exit option and identify an exit strategy, such as discontinuing routine medications to shorten the dying process.[46] Creating a vision of a peaceful, pain-free death is the first step in avoiding endless and frequently painful medical treatments.

Harrington writes exit strategies cover such conditions as "sepsis, the respiratory failure of pneumonia (with morphine for comfort), a sudden arrhythmia, dehydration, low blood sugar, or a metabolically induced coma."[47] Of course, delirium, seizures, uncontrollable pain, hallucinations, extreme agitation, feelings of despair, and other scary symptoms might still happen even for a patient with an exit strategy. Harrington writes, "Even under the best circumstances, the process of dying is messy, intense, unappealing, and unpredictable."[48] However, having an exit strategy significantly increases the chances of a peaceful and dignified death characterized by control, comfort, acceptance, and loving goodbyes.

* * * * *

This chapter has been about thinking through what we want at the end of life, creating advance directives, and having what author Dr. Atul Gawande calls "the hard conversation." Having that conversation, preparing an advance directive, and finding (and talking with) a health-care agent are all ways to tell your loved ones what you want at the end of your life. This is crucial to achieving a good death. But there is more they need to know, and this is encapsulated in a legacy letter (also called an ethical will) and in your memoirs—the subjects of the next chapter.

CHAPTER 5

Legacy Letters, Ethical Wills, and Memoirs

LEGACY COMES IN TWO BROAD FORMS. THE FIRST COVERS NONMONE-tary things like stories, journals, letters, and memoirs. The second covers monetary items such as money and possessions. This chapter focuses on the part of our legacy that's nonmonetary. We want to pass on our values and life lessons because they constitute the memories that will keep us alive in the hearts of those we leave behind. We live on after we die in our legacy. When we are no longer here, our friends and family can find us in our children, grandchildren, nephews, and nieces.

Historian Doris Kearns Goodwin wrote that Eleanor Roosevelt often quoted the lines, "They are not dead who live in lives they leave behind. In those whom they have blessed, they live a life again." In other words, after we die, we can live in others by what we gave. This is why it can be so beneficial to write a memoir, a goodbye letter, a life review letter, a legacy letter, an ethical will, a witness statement, or a personal mission statement—so our loved ones know what is deep in our heart. These similar and interconnected documents, filled with our values and most profound thoughts, can strengthen family bonds even after we die. They link the living with the dead.

At the end of life, we want to feel our life is complete. No one wants open loops and unfinished business—relationships raw and bruised, issues unresolved, projects unfinished, or love unexpressed. We also want to be able to give a coherent answer to two questions: What did my life mean? And did my life matter? One way to answer these profound and probing questions is to tell stories that bring coherence and meaning to all the events and activities that fill our lives.

Leaving a legacy means leaving our knowledge and wisdom for future generations. It involves discovering what it is about ourselves that we value and think is worth preserving. A legacy is built through conversations with loved ones, storytelling, modeling admirable behavior, and interactions with others. It is also built through writing. Putting our hard-earned life lessons and wisdom in writing—in the form, for example, of legacy letters, ethical wills, and memoirs—is an essential component of being able to die well.

Softening the Sting of Death

We die twice: first, when our bodies perish and, second, when our names are no longer mentioned and we become forgotten. Legacy letters (also called ethical wills) and memoirs soften the sting of both deaths. They give us peace of mind as death comes closer. We are likelier to have a good death if we have written a legacy letter and a memoir because we will have a sense of completion and fulfillment.

In chapter 2, I wrote that people fear death partly because "it means the end of our relationship with those we love and cherish." But that need not happen. Death does *not* mean the end of our relationship with the deceased. It's possible, in a way, to "talk" to the dead by reading their legacy letters and memoirs.

We want to create a meaningful legacy that will survive us and be our gift to the future. We want our memory "to be for a blessing," as the beautiful Jewish saying goes. We want to leave more than just money and possessions. We want to "ripple" into the future and enlarge the lives of others who survive us.[1] Creating a legacy letter (or recording) is one way to do that. Business strategist Peter Strople writes, "Legacy is not leaving something *for* people. It's leaving something *in* people."[2] And psychologist Erik Erikson writes, "I am what survives me."[3]

Responsibility to Those We Leave Behind

Our fear of death is diminished when we leave good works behind and live on in the lives of our loved ones and family. There are many forms such good works can take, ranging from legacy letters, to creating enduring nonprofits, to helping grandchildren flourish. They all help to ameliorate death by leaving behind something survivors will treasure. After we die, we want to be considered a farsighted and wise ancestor. Our death does not end our responsibility to those we leave behind. We want to be a light that shines through our family and friends for generations. We can support our loved ones even after we have died.

"Toast" Letters

When the pandemic began in March 2020, I started writing warm and heartfelt letters of appreciation and thanks to family members and good friends because I wanted them to know I loved and treasured them. These letters were "eulogies for the living" for the people I love. I called them "toast" letters because I was toasting them, and I included, for a touch of humor, an image of a piece of toast alongside a picture of a glass of champagne.[4]

The reason for the "toast" letters was simple: I wanted to express my love and appreciation to the people who had given me so much, supported me so generously, loved me despite my faults, and made a positive difference in my life. Writing my "toast" letters gave me enormous pleasure, and the letters gave joy to those who received them, especially because they were not expecting them. It's powerful to feel fully appreciated by the people closest to you. I spoke from my heart, even though I had to overcome the occasional feelings of awkwardness. I was not accustomed to expressing myself so openly.

In our society, we wait too long to recognize and honor the gifts and attributes of those we love. We often save compliments and words of admiration for after they have died, when they can no longer hear and cherish them. Instead, we should write "eulogies for the living" to our loved ones and friends, allowing us to connect and communicate on a deeper level while we are alive. My "toast" letters reminded friends and family that I cared about them, loved them, and that they had gifts and strengths I appreciated and valued. The letters took a lot of time, but I consider them an excellent investment in building relationships. Appendix II shows one of my toast letters.

Any day could be my last, so getting those letters done while I am still strong and healthy enough to do them helps give me a sense of completeness (and thus peace). In my book *Finding Meaning and Success*, I wrote about the desirability of having as few regrets as possible when dying. My "toast" letters reduced the potential regret on my deathbed of not having told my family and friends that I love them.

LEGACY LETTERS

Another way of telling your family and friends you love them is to prepare a legacy letter, also known as an ethical will. Ethical wills, legal wills, and living wills are all wills, but they have little in common. *Ethical wills* (legacy letters) focus on your values; *legal wills* focus on your estate, money, and assets; and *living wills* (also known as advance directives) focus on your health-care agent and end-of-life wishes.

The idea behind creating a legacy letter is to capture your essence as a person and your vision for the future so that future generations (your heirs) can benefit. In this way, you can support your family even after you are gone. A legacy letter transmits your nonmonetary "stuff" (your values, beliefs, stories, life lessons, and wisdom) to your loved ones. It attempts to answer some deep questions: What do you want your loved ones to know about the life you have led? What have you learned that's worth passing on? What are your values, and why do they matter to you? How did you find meaning and purpose in your life? What is the best way to live a good life?

Legacy letters grew out of a Jewish custom that originated many centuries ago. Older Jewish parents wrote letters that expressed their love and shared their wisdom and advice. They highlighted vital life lessons and described the lives they hoped their children might lead. Those letters came to be known as "ethical wills" or "legacy letters." Many people desire to pass on what is important to future generations. Your legacy letter helps to capture your character and spirit, articulates what's important to you, and contains stories you want remembered. Rabbi Steve Leder writes that a legacy letter is "the greatest gift one can give or receive. It is the most precious treasure we can pass on."[5]

A legacy letter summarizes what you've learned from life so it's not forgotten when you die. It expresses your love and gratitude to those you love who survive you. It attempts to answer the question, What did you create or contribute during, in poet Mary Oliver's phrasing, your "one wild and precious life"?[6]

Your legacy letter is a chance to express love, say thank you, ask for and grant forgiveness, and say goodbye—the five life tasks identified by palliative care doctor Ira Byock as things we should strive to accomplish. Loving, thoughtful older people create legacy letters to produce an enduring message. They are a recognition that, whatever physical or financial assets we may have, our most significant wealth is our love, values, stories, wisdom, guidance, and vision for the future.

Composing a Legacy Letter

Composing a legacy letter is a profoundly satisfying experience. It helps preserve your memory and gives you, the author, a fulfilling sense of completion and peace. A legacy letter need not be long; two to five pages is reasonable. Nor do you need to wait until your death to share it with your loved ones. On the contrary, sharing a draft as you write the letter may open up deep and meaningful conversations.

Your loved ones receive inspiration, comfort, love, and guidance and gain a more transparent window into the unique person you are. Legacy letters are a way to pass on your hopes for future generations and what you would like them to know about you. Writing a legacy letter is not easy. It's challenging to be introspective and reflective and look deeply into yourself for insights and wisdom. However, the following three steps can help make the task less onerous: Determine your audience and goals, brainstorm ideas, and write a first draft.

Your Audience and Goals

You may want to write more than one legacy letter. For example, you may want to write one to your children, another to your grandchildren, and perhaps a third to your siblings. On the other hand, some people write a single legacy letter addressed to their heirs and other loved ones. Your relationships and hope for a meaningful connection will help you decide whether to write more than one letter.

Once you've determined your audience, you will want to clarify your goals. They will likely include sharing life lessons, saying what's important to you, and describing your values (perhaps told through pertinent stories from your life). Your goals probably will include outlining your hopes for the future and expressing your love and gratitude.

BRAINSTORM IDEAS

Now is the time to begin jotting down your thoughts on what you might want to say about your life story, your values, what gives your life purpose, your feelings toward those you love and treasure, and your hopes for their future. You must find the words that express your love and gratitude toward your loved ones and what they mean to you. Reflect on what you want them to feel when they read your legacy letter. What do you cherish about them? How did they enrich your life? What hopes do you have for their future? Do you need to forgive them for anything? Do you need to *ask* for forgiveness? What do you need to thank them for? Can you tell them, "I love you"?

You may also want to brainstorm about any significant projects, roles, or commitments you were involved in, why they mattered, and how they gave your life meaning. How did those obligations and responsibilities embody and reflect the values by which you lived your life? Such values might include tenacity, generosity, self-discipline, creativity, frugality, or service. They might involve issues or causes such as protecting the environment, fighting injustice, helping people experiencing homelessness, or fostering education.

Another area to brainstorm is your philosophy of life. What guiding principles shepherded you through diverse life experiences, some of which were undoubtedly painful, stressful, and challenging? Reflect on what practical advice and wisdom you can offer. Those reading your legacy letter will appreciate receiving your counsel on important issues relating to children, love, friendship, marriage, success, work, career, health, social media, and other things related to the quality of life.

Writing a First Draft

Now is the time to review the accumulated notes from brainstorming and draft your legacy letter. Writing something down is essential so you can begin editing and improving the document. Your legacy letter is a work in progress. It is perfectly acceptable to produce a less-than-perfect first draft. It is far better to have an imperfect first draft than a blank sheet of paper.

Write from the heart and convey that your life has value; one reason for this is your relationship with your family, loved ones, and friends. Share how important these special people are to you. Doing so may strengthen your relationships with the people who most matter to you. In writing your legacy letter, you will have done your best to provide future generations with a valuable gift, something they may cherish and view with pride, reverence, and gratitude as an enduring example of your spirit and character. Examples of legacy letters can be found by searching "legacy letters and ethical wills" on the Internet. You can find three of my legacy letters in appendix II.

Reread your first draft to ensure it is not preachy or pushy. Your readers want to be informed about you and your values and to be able to incorporate what is meaningful to them in their own lives without feeling guilty about the choices they make for themselves. You might even want to touch on errors or mistakes you committed that you'd like your loved ones to learn from and, hopefully, avoid. If talking about your blunders and stumbles is too painful, you could write about one or two of the lesser struggles in your life and how you overcame setbacks and disappointments. Relaying your successes and triumphs is also essential, especially when you can use those stories to illustrate when you were at your best and exhibited tenacity, humility, altruism, and compassion.

Stanford University's Life-Review Letter Project

Geriatrician and palliative care doctor VJ Periyakoil at the Stanford University Medical Center has developed a project similar to a legacy letter. She says that the most common emotion among dying patients is regret. To deal with this, she encourages her patients to write a life-review letter to their loved ones. Periyakoil's project has grown into the Stanford

Friends and Family Letter Project, which provides a free template for a letter that can help people complete several life-review tasks: acknowledging important people in our lives; remembering treasured moments; apologizing to those we might have hurt; forgiving those who have hurt us; and saying "thank you," "I love you," and "goodbye." You can find the letter template at med.stanford.edu/letter.

Sadly, many people don't complete these steps before they die, leaving their surviving loved ones with unanswered questions, sadness, and regrets. As with a legacy letter, writing a life-review letter takes courage because it can bring discomfort and vexing feelings. But it may be the most important letter you will ever write because it tells your loved ones that they matter to you and that you love them totally and unconditionally.

MEMOIR OR AUTOBIOGRAPHY

Another way to express your love for your survivors is to write a memoir. Memoirs and autobiographies are often confused, but there is a distinction. Both are stories of someone's life written by that person and in the first person. In a memoir, the author shares memories from a specific period or reflects upon a theme or a particular facet of her life. In contrast, an autobiography is an account of the author's entire life. I will use the word *memoir*, but my comments below apply to autobiographies too.

When you contemplate the brevity of your life, one thing you may fear is that you have no future. Another fear is that your past life, memories, and experiences will vanish. Writing a memoir can help to assuage that fear. It allows you to tell the unique story of how you came to be who you are and describe the events, relationships, crises, triumphs, setbacks, and experiences that shaped you. Giving your loved ones and future generations the story of your fully lived life is a sublime gift.

A memoir is a record of your life. Unless you document your personal family history, it will likely be lost, forgotten, and untold. When you write a memoir, you create something meaningful and important. It can be as short as two pages, or it can be book length. You are making a legacy project that will enrich the lives of your loved ones. Viewing life experiences, both joyful and traumatic, through the prism of leaving a legacy can help you discover new meanings in events and happenings you have experienced. Parents and their adult children often have different views of the parent's legacy. They might not know each other as well as they think. A memoir's value is that it can bring greater understanding between the generations.[7]

When writing a memoir, the first thing to do is to start a creative journal. A creative journal is a notebook, ideally with the pages lined and numbered, to facilitate organizing and tracking information. Whenever you think of an idea for your memoir, jot it down in the journal. Your creative journal is a safe, private place to capture memories and experiment with different ideas for structuring your memoir.

A Good Memoir

Many things make a good memoir, including the following:

1. Telling the good and the bad (so your memoir isn't misleadingly idyllic);

2. Being gracious when writing about others (i.e., using discretion);

3. Authenticity and being yourself;

4. Telling stories; and

5. Writing with your audience in mind (your grandchildren? siblings? the general public? a particular demographic?).

An important question to ponder is *why* do you want to write a memoir? The "why" keeps you going when you hit obstacles or lose motivation or momentum. In his famous book *Man's Search for Meaning*, Viktor Frankl wrote that a person can bear any "how" if he has a "why." So, when you get stuck writing your memoir, keep returning to the "why."

Many people who write a memoir get overwhelmed by the massiveness of the job. The way to deal with this is to break the project down into tasks and subtasks. There are several ways to do that. You can create chapters by dividing your life by decades. Or divide your life by pivotal events. Or divide your life by significant decisions you've made. Or list how your goals changed as you moved through life. Or divide your life by the central stepping-stones in a relationship. There are many other ways to divide the work and make it more manageable. I organized one of my memoirs around confessions and mistakes I had made.

Memoirs are more fun and exciting to read if they contain stories. Stories create an emotional connection and help make the information more memorable. Readers gain a deeper understanding of other people's lives through stories. Because stories are engaging (in a way that pure facts and figures are not), readers are likelier to take in the message and its meaning.

The three essential elements of a story are the following:

1. Taking a journey: an initiating incident, problem, or desire;

2. Facing a challenge: struggles with adversity, disappointments, and setbacks;

3. Finding a victory: crisis, climax, realization, or transformation.

AN EXERCISE IN REMEMBERING

You may be worried that you can't remember the details of events and experiences. An exercise in remembering is to think of an experience you want to include in your memoir. Close your eyes. Breathe deeply. Imagine yourself living through the incident again. Then, open your eyes and write in your creative journal, describing what you see, hear, and feel.

Another helpful exercise is to choose a moment you don't remember well and write about it in the present tense. Any memory fragment will do. For example, your earliest memory, an embarrassing moment, or an experience that took your breath away. Write fast, don't stop, and don't worry about spelling or good English. This technique can sometimes help blast through memory blocks as you are writing.

Two additional ways to trigger and spark memories you may have forgotten or repressed are looking at old photos and building "a memory house." Old photos can remind you of long-forgotten stories. To build "a memory house," get a piece of paper and draw a floor plan of a home where you lived. Then, slowly go through the house, letting it trigger memories, and write them down in your journal in as much detail as possible.

StoryWorth

If writing a memoir still seems intimidating and overwhelming, an easier approach is to use the services of a company called StoryWorth. My oldest daughter Kimberly gave my wife and me StoryWorth for a year. Every week, we received a question carefully curated by Kimberly and had one week to answer it. We did this as thoughtfully and conscientiously as we could for a year. At year's end, StoryWorth compiled our answers into a 320-page book as a legacy gift. The website for StoryWorth is www .storyworth.com.

* * * * *

We write legacy letters, ethical wills, and memoirs for our surviving loved ones. Often, those people are also our caregivers at the end of our lives. A lot more needs to be done for caregivers. That's the topic of the next chapter.

Chapter 6

Caring for Caregivers

CAREGIVERS SUPPORT PEOPLE WHO NEED HELP TAKING CARE OF THEM-selves. Those needing help may require assistance because of illness, surgery, frailty, or for other reasons.[1] Unfortunately, many caregivers neglect their own well-being. This chapter examines caregivers, what they experience, and how they suffer. It also looks at what can be done to alleviate their suffering.

More than fifty-three million adults in the United States are caregivers—more than one in four adults or about one sixth of the population.[2,3] They perform unpaid family caregiving and manage the physical, emotional, and social needs of loved ones in need. They are vastly underappreciated.

Caring for a sick and dying person is exhausting and often thankless work. The patient may show little or no appreciation for all the help that's being provided. Perhaps that's because the patient is struggling to stay alive against the insidious intrusion into his body of whatever condition is afflicting him. Thus, the person needing help may be oblivious to the stress and fatigue of the caregiver.

NOT ENOUGH CAREGIVERS

According to AARP, nearly 70 percent of Americans who reach sixty-five will someday require assistance from others to get through the day.[4] Unfortunately, few of us want to face up to this fact because few admit that we or our loved ones will decline at some point and become a burden on others.[5]

The problem is that the way America provides long-term care to those who need it due to disease, dementia, or old age is, says AARP, "deeply flawed."[6] Wealthy people have the money to buy the care they need, and people without resources have Medicaid, but there is a colossal number of people between these two extremes who are essentially on their own and need the assistance of unpaid family caregivers. (The shortcomings and challenges of nursing homes are a related but separate problem beyond the focus of this book.)

The brutal truth is that we do not have enough caregivers for the current number of older Americans.[7] We have also created a situation where those providing the most intimate care to older people are, in author and gerontologist Tracey Gendron's words, "overworked, underpaid, unsupported, and unrecognized."[8]

CAREGIVING IS HARD

Providing caregiving to a dying person is a new experience for many caregivers and a scary one. Caregivers know their loved one will die, and they worry about making mistakes and unintentionally hurting the person. They also worry about what will happen when death comes. What will dying and death look like? And they suffer anticipatory grief (more on grief in chapter 12).

It's true that the experience can also be sacred and even transcendent despite the job's unpleasant parts. Ultimately, caregiving can be profoundly fulfilling and memorable. However exhausting and vexing caregiving can be, caregivers will likely look back on the experience as deeply rewarding and important and a time when they were at their most honorable, decent, and giving.

That said, caregiving is often intensely demanding and burdensome, with days and nights full of changing dirty diapers, giving pills and medications, administering intravenous antibiotics, managing finances, and doing other tedious and exhausting jobs. Prolonged debility and longevity of the patient exacerbate all this. Caregiving is often mind-numbing, exhausting, uncomfortably intimate, and sometimes distasteful (for example, when inserting pills rectally or dealing with bedsores or other foul-smelling wounds).

The job includes running errands, preparing meals, loading the dishwasher, grocery shopping, driving the patient to doctor appointments, doing laundry, changing diapers, cleaning up vomit, bathing the patient, dressing wounds, grooming the patient, and doing all this while frequently having to accept a hurtful lack of appreciation and gratitude. The recognition offered for all the caregiving is often minuscule and insignificant.

Caregiving is also a risky enterprise. Lifting a patient on and off a toilet and into and out of bed can lead to back injuries and torn muscles. Caregivers are at increased risk for anxiety and stress. One way to reduce the stress is for patients to be grateful to them and express that gratitude regularly. You can be surprisingly frail yet still be able to offer encouragement, praise, and appreciation to someone lovingly taking care of you.

Everyone Must Help

When a person is coming to the end of life and wants to have a good death, then loved ones and friends of the dying person have a vital role to play. When a family gathers around a person with limited time left, that family has an opportunity to strengthen the relationship of its members, providing that the caregiving tasks are shared equally and no family member gets exhausted or burned out.

All the grown children of aging parents should play a role in looking after Mom and Dad. However, a study by Northwestern Mutual found that the responsibility for caregiving most likely falls on the shoulders of one sibling.[9] That's not fair. If one child handles the parents' care, others can do needed online research into medications, take care of home repairs and maintenance, manage the bills, or give the primary caregiver a regular respite. This way, all can have a clear conscience, knowing they pulled their weight and did their fair share. One thing that can exacerbate grief after a person has died is the guilt that we didn't do enough to help.

Most caregivers are female, and nearly all are related to the patient.[10] That is incredibly unfair. It's not uncommon for a daughter to take on most of the caregiving for aging parents while the sons contribute little.

In this circumstance, where one family member is taking on a disproportionate share of the caregiving burden, I recommend paying her a decent hourly wage (if possible) and being transparent about it by letting other family members know of this.

CAREGIVER SELF-CARE

Caregiving may involve meeting complex demands without any training or help. It may also require juggling the caregiving responsibilities with holding down a job or taking care of children or others. It's not uncommon for caregivers to put their needs and feelings aside to meet all of the demands. But that's not good for their long-term health.

Being a capable and reliable caregiver means giving a high priority to taking care of yourself. You need to do so to have the strength and ability to care for your loved one. A few things that will help include reaching out for palliative and hospice care and finding someone to take your place for a short period to give you a break. Do meditation, yoga, journaling, or anything to give yourself some love during that respite. And reach out to friends for support or someone who will listen to you vent.

CAREGIVER STRESS

For untrained caregivers, which means most family members, looking after a dying loved one can be overwhelming, even with hospice care. What if the patient falls? What if the person starts bleeding or becomes delirious or agitated? What if the patient suffers acute, agonizing pain?

According to the Office on Women's Health in the US Department of Health and Human Services, caregiver stress affects many caregivers. This stress comes from the emotional and physical strain of caregiving.[11] The signs include the following:

1. Feeling overwhelmed

2. Feeling alone, isolated, or deserted by others

3. Sleeping too much or too little

4. Gaining or losing a lot of weight

5. Feeling tired most of the time

6. Losing interest in activities you used to enjoy

7. Becoming easily irritated or angered

8. Feeling worried or sad often

9. Having headaches or body aches often

10. Turning to unhealthy behaviors, such as smoking or drinking too much alcohol

Long-term caregiver stress may put you at risk for many health problems. Some of these problems can be serious. They include the following:

1. Anxiety and depression

2. A weak immune system

3. Excess weight

4. Chronic diseases, such as heart disease, cancer, and diabetes

Taking steps to relieve caregiver stress may help prevent health problems. Remember that you can provide better care for your loved one if you feel healthy. It will also be easier to focus on the rewards of caregiving. Some ways to help yourself include the following:

1. Learning better ways to help your loved one. For example, hospitals offer classes that can teach you how to care for someone with an injury or illness.

2. Finding caregiving resources in your community. Many communities have adult daycare services or respite services. Using one of these can give you a break from your caregiving duties.

3. Asking for and accepting help. Make a list of ways others can help you. Let helpers choose what they would like to do. For instance,

someone might sit with the person you care for while you do an errand. Someone else might pick up groceries for you.

4. Joining a support group for caregivers. A support group can allow you to share stories, pick up caregiving tips, and get support from others who face your challenges.

5. Being organized. This makes caregiving more manageable. Make to-do lists and set a daily routine.

6. Staying in touch with family and friends. You need to have emotional support.

7. Taking care of your own health. Try to find time to exercise most days of the week, choose healthy foods, and get sufficient sleep. In addition, make sure that you keep up with your medical care, including screenings and regular checkups.

8. Consider taking a break from your job if you also work and feel overwhelmed. Under the federal Family and Medical Leave Act, eligible employees can take up to twelve weeks of unpaid leave per year to care for relatives. Check with your human resources office about available options.

SEAGULL RELATIVES

As families gather around a sick patient, resentments and other festering emotional wounds can bloom toxically.

Some members of the family who are closest to the dying loved one and know him best (and have been the most devoted caregivers in the family) will likely say, "Let Grandpa die naturally and peacefully." In contrast, other family members, perhaps those who have been distant and neglectful, will demand that the doctors "do everything to save him."

Arguments and fights can easily break out, especially if the patient has failed to complete an advance directive and left no guidance on his wants. An advance directive is a profound gift to your family because it can spare a family much gratuitous contention and strife.

Author and cardiologist Dr. Haider Warraich defines the "seagull" relative as the "distant and remote relative who seems to fly in only when the situation couldn't be more acute and, in many cases, brings a completely new and different perspective to the situation." Warraich quotes CrashingPatient.com as saying, "They fly in, crap on everything, and fly away." He adds that guilt is a characteristic often demonstrated by seagulls. Many feel bad that they have neglected the patient, and their remorse transforms into an overzealous desire to "save" the patient.[12] The patient's wishes must be given precedence over the demands of a "seagull" relative who is out to metaphorically defecate on others in the family who are doing their best for the patient.

WHAT NOT TO SAY

Unfortunately, not all caregivers are benign in tense and fraught situations. When they are exhausted and feel unappreciated, it is easy for them to let good judgment slip and say the wrong thing to the person cared for. For example, it's best not to talk about your religious beliefs unless you are sure the patient agrees with them. It's best not to admonish the patient not to give up and argue that he will beat the illness. And it's probably not helpful to talk about another patient's suffering and try to draw lessons from that.

English-American author and journalist Christopher Hitchens told the story in his book *Mortality* of a woman he never knew who said to him as he died of esophageal cancer, "I just want you to know that I understand *exactly* what you are going through."[13] But nobody can honestly make that claim, and Hitchens points out that choosing your words carefully when talking to a severely sick or dying person is important.

Don't say, "Everything happens for a reason," "God is trying to get you to listen," "You need a good attitude to survive," or "Everything will be okay." Instead, listen intently, and, when you do talk, say things like, "I love you," "I'm here for you," and "Is there anything you'd like to talk about?" People trying to be supportive often say to a sick person, "Let me know how I can help." However, experts in illness etiquette, like author Steven Petrow, say it is better to offer something specific: to walk their dog, wash up, bring a meal, or do the laundry.[14]

* * * * *

This chapter has focused on the plight of caregivers. It is a major problem that will only worsen as Baby Boomers swell the ranks of the aging and frail. But palliative care, hospice, and death doulas can help as the end of life approaches. Those are the topics of the next chapter.

CHAPTER 7

Palliative Care, Hospice, and End-of-Life Doulas

IN THE 1980S, PALLIATIVE CARE AND HOSPICE WERE NEW IDEAS STRUG-gling to get recognition as standard medical care. Now, they are well established but still not used enough. This chapter explores the benefits of palliative care, hospice, and end-of-life doulas and the necessary vigilance to get the most out of these essential services.

Most of us in the United States will die of chronic diseases in old age, and many illnesses cause a slow decline toward death over months or years. As life winds down, we need to rely more on gentler medical interventions, such as palliative care, to support a good quality of life. Palliative care is specialized medical care for people living with a serious illness. It relieves the symptoms and stress of diseases like cancer, demen-tia, lung disease, kidney failure, and heart disease, whether the suffering is physical, emotional, social, or spiritual.

PALLIATIVE CARE

Palliative care can be provided to patients simultaneously as they receive curative treatment for a serious illness. They don't have to wait until their disease is advanced to start palliative care. This care can be used at any time after the diagnosis. Patients can request palliative care consultations at diagnosis or during worsening symptoms. It doesn't focus on curing the disease (the responsibility of other doctors) but instead on easing suf-fering and improving the quality of life. Palliative care doctors know that quality of life is important and sometimes more important to patients than trying to prolong life indefinitely.

When facing a relentless disease, palliative care is invaluable; the earlier a patient gets help, the better. Palliative care doctors help manage anxiety, agitation, nausea, constipation, fatigue, and air hunger. They work side-by-side with the doctors whose aim is to cure illness and prolong life. Palliative care doctors focus on the whole patient and family members with support rooted in kindness, respect, and compassion. They encourage patients to be fully in charge of their own care and make decisions consistent with their values and preferences. Palliative care is a response to the hyperspecialization and fragmentation of health care in which doctors tend to specialize in a specific organ, such as the heart or kidneys. In contrast, palliative care doctors see patients as far more than an assemblage of organs.

Palliative care generally is based in hospices, hospitals, nursing homes, and outpatient palliative care clinics or occurs at home. A palliative care team may include specialist nurses and doctors, social workers, religious or spiritual leaders, therapists, or nutritionists, among other professionals. The team will vary depending on the needs of the patient. The Center to Advance Palliative Care (CAPC) offers resources to identify palliative care services in different localities; find them at https://getpalliativecare .org/.

Studies have shown that palliative care can have many benefits for both patients and their families. Those enrolled in palliative care have fewer symptoms, greater emotional support, and increased patient and family satisfaction.[1] Research has shown that palliative care helps terminally ill patients, even while those patients are pursuing aggressive cures. They live longer and have improved quality of life compared to those patients who neglect to seek palliative care.

Many patients fear the trauma of physical pain more than the fear of dying. Palliative care physician Dr. Jessica Zitter writes, "Statistics show that increasing numbers of people are dying in pain, according to their surrogates: 61 percent in 2014, a 12 percent leap from 1998."[2] The good news is that many studies show that palliative care can mitigate pain and give relief.

Hospice Care

Hospice care is a specialized form of palliative care delivered to patients with a life expectancy of six months or less.[3] By this time, trying to cure the disease is no longer an option, so efforts to cure are replaced by comfort care. Hospices provide a way to focus on optimizing the quality of life for those nearing death. According to the National Hospice and Palliative Care Organization (NHPCO), 1.61 million Medicare beneficiaries received hospice care in 2019. This represents a considerable increase over 2000 (529,573) and 2010 (1.2 million).[4]

Hospice is a philosophy of care that uses palliative care principles with terminally ill patients. Unfortunately, some doctors believe that using hospice means they have failed, and, to some patients, using hospice represents giving up. Both suppositions are wrong. Many studies have shown that patients with serious diseases underutilize hospice and palliative care. Doctors and patients need to be educated about the benefits of these two resources and encouraged to use them more. Research shows that patients seek out hospice too late, and doctors wait too long to refer their patients to hospice. When a dying loved one is in hospice, many families say, "I wish we had started hospice earlier." Unfortunately, most people don't receive hospice care until the final weeks or even days of life, missing out on months of helpful care and quality time.

As Dr. BJ Miller and Shoshana Berger write, "It is rarely too early to enroll" with hospice.[5] Similarly, hospice and palliative care physician Dr. Sunita Puri writes, "Many of the patients I see die within a few days or weeks (of starting hospice), never fully enjoying the benefits of the care we try to provide."[6]

Both palliative and hospice care are designed to relieve suffering, optimize quality of life, and help patients live well until they die. Both can help people live longer with less stress and anxiety and more comfort. Hospice pioneer Dame Cicely Saunders from Great Britain first introduced the idea of specialized care for the dying to the United States in a lecture at Yale University in 1963. She founded the first modern hospice in London, St. Christopher's, in 1967. St. Christopher's is a residential facility for dying patients. Saunders told her patients, "You matter to the last moment of your life, and we will do all we can, not only to help you die peacefully but to live until you die."[7]

In the United States, hospice does not refer to a place or an organization but to a type of care that gently comforts a terminally ill person. Hospice in the United States is carried out primarily in people's homes. Hospice-care services are generally covered in full by Medicare and most other insurances.[8] To qualify for hospice care, you must have a terminal disease (one that will result in your death) and a doctor's assessment that you will most likely die within six months. Inpatient hospices are the exception in the United States but are a godsend when caring for a patient at home becomes too demanding and the patient needs hospital-level acute care, such as intravenous medications.[9]

Trading a lower quality of life for a greater quantity of life (extending life at all costs) leads to overmedicalization for older patients. Hospice reverses this process. It focuses on the whole person at the end of life and improves the quality of life while the terminal disease takes its natural course.[10] Author and surgeon Dr. Atul Gawande writes, "You don't have to spend much time with the elderly or those with a terminal illness to see how often medicine fails the people it is supposed to help." He says that, toward the end of their lives, patients are given treatments that addle their brains and sap their bodies for zero or negligible benefits.[11]

As the end of life draws closer, medical interventions usually rise. For example, a third of older Americans undergo a surgical procedure in the hospital in the last year of life.[12] According to cardiologist Dr. Haider Warraich, 20 percent of patients undergo life-sustaining interventions such as intubation, CPR, and artificial nutrition in the last six months of life.[13] Such interventions might not provide benefits when performed so close to dying.

HOSPICE MULTIDISCIPLINARY TEAMS AND COMPLEMENTARY INTERVENTIONS

Hospice care is used when patients and their families no longer wish to pursue treatments meant to slow or halt the progression of an illness and instead want to focus on comfort and the reduction of suffering. As noted, most hospice care in the United States occurs in the patient's home (or wherever the patient lives), where people are allowed to die naturally with loved ones surrounding them. In a crisis, loved ones should call the hospice before calling 911 because hospice aims to treat agitation or other problems at home and avoid getting on the "conveyor belt" of treatments in the hospital.[14]

Hospice care aims to manage pain and suffering so that patients can thrive at the end of their lives as best they can. It also helps patients—and their loved ones and caregivers—not only physically but also emotionally and spiritually. This is possible because a hospice interdisciplinary team includes doctors, nurses, social workers, hospice aides, interfaith chaplains, trained volunteers, bereavement counselors, and complementary therapists. Together, they offer a wide range of services.

They can provide medical supplies and equipment, respite services (relief for the caregiver), medications to manage pain and other symptoms, and spiritual support. The supplies and medical equipment often include an adjustable hospital bed, a wheelchair, a bedside toilet, and needed drugs and medications. Visits by trained volunteers are offered regularly, and 24/7 telephone support is always available. When a patient starts to die actively, hospice nurse visits occur more frequently to help the family and change medications as needed.

Many hospices, especially nonprofit ones, offer complementary or nonpharmacological interventions (as an adjunct to conventional treatment), including touch (such as hand massages with lavender), music therapy, art therapy, pet companionship, and aromatherapy.

How Hospice Helps

Ironically, studies show that older patients in hospice can live longer than similar patients who select surgery and other medical interventions. In other words, choosing hospice over continuing curative care can sometimes extend a patient's life. Moreover, hospice and comfort care increase the chances of a peaceful death. In contrast, endlessly seeking treatment almost certainly results in a painful medicalized death in an intensive-care unit. Dr. Samuel Harrington writes, "Blessed are the frail elderly who do not have to visit the emergency room."[15]

Many people assume that hospice hastens death because a patient gives up seeking a cure, but, as just noted, the evidence from multiple studies shows that hospice can extend life.[16] Author and activist Barbara Coombs Lee writes, "Groups of cancer and heart disease patients enrolled in hospice or receiving palliative care services live longer, on average, than patients who receive only treatments to fight their disease and none to ensure their comfort."[17]

Gawande cites a remarkable 2010 study from the Massachusetts General Hospital. It found that cancer patients who saw a palliative care specialist "stopped chemotherapy sooner, entered hospice far earlier, experienced less suffering at the end of their lives—*and they lived 25 percent longer.*"[18] (The italics are in the original.) Gawande's point is that modern medicine is "actively inflicting harm on patients rather than confronting the subject of mortality."[19]

The benefits of hospice care include the following:

1. Increasing the likelihood of a person dying at home

2. Offering dignity and calm, especially compared to dying in a hospital, which can often be busy, noisy, and disturbing

3. Possibly extending a patient's life

4. Preventing expensive and often inhumane hospitalizations and ICU admissions just before a patient dies

5. Offering grief and bereavement counseling

Hospice is not a fast track to death. Patients are not giving up on life. They are simply choosing a smoother, gentler ride for the journey and living their best life until they die.

FOR-PROFIT VERSUS NONPROFIT HOSPICES

Hospices can be either nonprofit or for profit. The data shows that, as a broad rule, nonprofit hospices perform better than for-profit ones, but as BJ Miller and Shoshana Berger write, "It's too simple to suggest for-profit enterprises are inherently bad, and nonprofits inherently good."[20]

For-profit hospices tend to be more problematic because they don't have the same mission as nonprofits. For-profits must make money, which can lead to cutting corners and a lack of care. Generating profit can occur at the expense of dying patients. Emergency-medicine physician and author Dan Morhaim writes, "I prefer nonprofit hospices as they generally are more concerned with patient care than profit."[21]

Similarly, author Dr. Sam Harrington says, "I generally prefer nonprofit hospices because they are more mission-driven than for-profit hospices."[22] Nonprofit hospices (full disclosure: I serve on the Board of the nonprofit Montgomery Hospice and Prince George's Hospice) set the gold standard for what a hospice should be—caring, humane, and gentle. The Government Accountability Office (GAO) has found that for-profit hospices are more likely than nonprofit hospices to have low rates of home visits in the last days of life.[23]

Hospice started in the United States in the late 1960s with small, volunteer-run organizations, but it has now transformed into a $20 billion industry with a radical increase in for-profit ownership. The rapid growth of for-profit hospices since 2000, especially when paired with the reduction in nonprofit hospices, is striking. For-profit hospices grew from 30 percent in 2000 to 71 percent in 2019. There were 672 for-profit hospices in 2000 and 3,437 by 2019. Nonprofit hospices decreased in number from 1,324 in 2000 to 1,248 in 2019.[24]

Put another way, in 2000, fewer than a third of hospices were for profit. By 2017, more than two-thirds of hospice providers were for profit. The number of hospices overall doubled, but the net increase was almost all in for-profit hospices. Today, for-profit hospices dominate the hospice market. The evidence that care quality is lower in for-profit hospices makes this ownership trend a cause for concern.

The ability to turn a quick profit in caring for people in their last days of life is attracting a new breed of hospice owners: private-equity firms. That has many hospice observers worried that the original hospice vision may be fading, as those capital investment companies' demand for return on investment is hurting patients and their families.

Many nonprofit hospices worry that private-equity–backed and other for-profit hospices are damaging the reputation of hospices generally. Author and playwright Margaret Engel writes,

> For-profit hospice can be good, but I know several cases where the pain meds weren't sufficient, and the families could not rouse hospice folks on nights and weekends to come back and up the dose. Several friends' loved ones suffered brutally under absent hospice caregiving. Several others hated giving the morphine themselves and believed they killed their loved ones because they upped the dose to keep them from agony, thrashing, and groaning.[25]

HOSPICE CAN'T DO EVERYTHING

Hospice care helps patients live fully until they die. So, in a real sense, hospice is about living, not dying. But while hospice teams are impressive, the fact remains that patients in hospice are on their own most of the time. There is abundant work left for friends and loved ones to do.

Hospice does not provide home care 24/7. You don't suddenly get a nursing-care team to take over when you get hospice care. Hospice team members provide house calls lasting one or two hours. Bathing, feeding, changing soiled diapers, and giving medication must be provided by loved ones or by aides hired and paid for by the family. The family continues to have to supply (or hire) home health-care aides.

The hospice nurse will teach caregivers how to administer medications, for example, morphine, if needed, but administering the medications is left to the family. Similarly, keeping the patient clean, changing bed sheets, shifting the patient's body to prevent bedsores, and a range of additional menial, tedious, and burdensome tasks are left for the family. If you can afford it, hiring a nursing or home health-care aide probably makes sense to help reduce the daily work burden on caregivers.

Hospice in the home is the best way to die and have a good death, assuming you want to die at home (most people do) and have loved ones or a network of relatives or friends to look after you or the resources to pay for hired caregivers. But not everyone has access to hospice, especially those outside urban areas.

WHERE TO DIE

For the first time since the early part of the twentieth century, more Americans are dying at home than in the hospital or a nursing home, and hospice is the primary reason.[26] It is tempting to assume that dying at home is always better than dying in a hospital, as it often is. Usually, being at home, surrounded by loved ones, will give you a better dying experience than being in a hospital, with tubes and machines everywhere.

But hospice and palliative-care physician Dr. Sunita Puri was surprised to discover that some of her patients preferred to die in a hospital because administering the proper medications can sometimes be too onerous a responsibility for loved ones caring for a patient growing agitated and delirious. The dying patient and the caregivers feel the patient should be in hospital under the watch of professionals who know how to administer the correct drugs at the proper levels.[27]

In a hospital, highly skilled nurses and doctors know precisely what needs to be done to alleviate pain in a way that a panicky, inexperienced caregiver at home might not. A peaceful death at home is not achievable for every dying patient. Dr. Puri writes,

> Fully experiencing the benefits of home hospice requires resources that hospice actually cannot provide: Money to afford caregivers, particularly in the absence of involved family members. A nearby pharmacy that stocks opiate medications for severe pain.[28]

Dying in a nursing home or hospital can be stressful because the patient often has to share a room with someone in the next bed, separated by a curtain. Under these circumstances, the family should ask the hospital or nursing home for a temporary private room. If one is available, that will help achieve a more peaceful death. Hopefully, every hospital will soon have "dying rooms," like "birthing rooms," where a dying person and the family can find peace, calm, and privacy.

Dying patients need, at a minimum, pain control, comfort, and love from family or friends, but even providing these basic things is occasionally too much for hospice care in the home. Sometimes, patients have to move from home hospice to hospice in a residential facility or hospital in the last days of life because they are too delirious, agitated, or have too much untreatable and uncontrolled pain to be cared for at home.[29] But, for the most part, patients are more likely to achieve a peaceful death with hospice in the home. Dying in a hospital can work well if the hospital is equipped with a hospice (or hospice-like) wing, but many are not.

In hospitals that are not set up in any way to let patients die peacefully (which is most of them), most die in an ICU, and those deaths can be anything but peaceful. This is because hospitals are designed to save lives, not achieve good deaths. As we've already noted, some doctors view death as a failure and thus may lose interest in dying patients and switch their attention to patients they can save.[30] Medical researcher Dr. Melissa Wachterman and her colleagues looked into the issue of the best place for patients to die (home, inpatient hospice facility, skilled nursing facility, hospitals, etc.) and concluded,

> For some patients and families, there's no place like home at the end of life; for others, a hospital, nursing facility, or inpatient hospice facility—where staff can manage symptoms and provide personal care, thereby enabling families to be families and maximize quality time together—may be the best place for a good death.[31]

END-OF-LIFE DOULAS

Many people are familiar with birth doulas, but "doula" is also used to describe people who help patients and families at the end of life. End-of-life doulas are sometimes called death midwives, end-of-life workers, or death doulas.

End-of-life doulas offer support, companionship, and guidance not only to the dying but also to partners, family members, and loved ones. They approach their work in a holistic manner, providing emotional, spiritual, and practical care, and are often central in helping the dying think about and develop a plan for how they would like to die. Doulas help to normalize the process of dying and grief by creating a space to hold skillfully guided conversations among the dying and loved ones, thereby increasing communication and supporting emotional and spiritual well-being.

If you can afford them, end-of-life doulas are often an excellent addition to hospice care because they can spend ample time with patients, coaching them, helping them emotionally, comforting them, listening to them, and keeping them physically comfortable and clean. End-of-life doulas can also help dying patients plan the end of their lives, collect ideas for their memorial service, incorporate traditions and rituals during the vigil process, take notes about their life stories, and even help them write letters to loved ones. And they provide respite for family members who are likely stressed and exhausted.[32]

End-of-life doulas are a wonderful supplement to hospice care because they provide the one thing hospice cannot, and that is spending virtually unlimited time with the families and patients. End-of-life doulas can be there at the time of death as well as before and afterward. Some volunteer their services, while others have full-time careers as death doulas.

Doulas may have a specialization. Some concentrate their services on remembrance and legacy work, while others may focus on the vigil process. Some may specialize in supporting patients who choose medical aid in dying.

End-of-life doulas can help provide some physical care (bathing, toileting, meal assistance, etc.), but this comes with a price tag that some families may be unable to afford. In contrast to hospice, the services of end-of-life doulas are not currently reimbursed by Medicare or insurance carriers. The dying patient or the family must pay for the end-of-life doula's services. Each doula will have a different arrangement, which should be discussed and negotiated. In the future, as we have seen in the field of birth doulas, insurance reimbursement and Medicare coverage could become possible in some states.

* * * * *

This chapter has explored how palliative care, hospice, and end-of-life doulas can be a godsend to patients seeking help dealing with severe illnesses and other potential end-of-life issues. However, as the end of life approaches, some patients want more agency over what is happening to them. This has fueled the death with dignity movement, which we will discuss in the next chapter.

CHAPTER 8

End-of-Life Options

DYING PEOPLE FACE THE PROSPECT OF PROLONGING LIFE AS LONG AS possible (and perhaps experiencing intolerable suffering and deterioration) or finding ways to die peacefully and gracefully. This chapter deals with a controversial issue: the right of an individual to choose how and when to end his life and how to have access to safe, caring, and legal means of doing so.

The "right to choose death" means that each individual should have the right to choose a peaceful, dignified death consistent with her values and to receive assistance in pursuing this right. People near death should be entitled to terminate their lives intentionally and deliberately, with dignity and support. The decision to hasten death is strictly an individual choice. This book is about giving people options at the end of life and letting them freely choose how they want to die.

Discussions about this are usually held with people with a serious progressive illness that may or may not be terminal but whose life has deteriorated so severely that quality of life has become (or soon will become) unacceptable and unbearable. For example, consider the author Cai Emmons, who died on January 2, 2023. Here is an excerpt from her final letter, written the day before:

Dear Friends and Readers,

. . . It is January 1st, 2023 and I am planning to depart from life as I've known it through death with dignity on January 2, 2023. I have had a rewarding life and I love everyone who has been a part of it. Remember me with joy.

. . . My body has become so weak that I have lost agency over my life and need help for most activities. We all have a line we draw in the sand regarding how much helplessness we can take, and I have reached mine.

DEATH IS NOT ALWAYS TO BE AGGRESSIVELY OPPOSED

In her book *Finish Strong: Putting Your Priorities First at Life's End*, Barbara Coombs Lee, a major figure in the movement for end-of-life choices and a long-time leader of the grassroots organization Compassion & Choices, tells the story of how she first began to understand that death is not always to be aggressively opposed. As a young nurse, Coombs Lee provided care to Ed, a patient with end-stage heart failure. She grew close to him and his wife over their months of hospital stays. Eventually, when Ed's heart went into fatal arrhythmia, Coombs Lee did as she was trained: She used the defibrillation paddles to shock Ed's heart, restoring him to a normal rhythm. To her surprise, Ed woke up angry and let Coombs Lee know it.

He had wanted to die peacefully and was livid that she had intervened without permission and prevented him from slipping quietly away. Coombs Lee suddenly realized that technological interventions are not always aligned with a person's priorities and values. Whatever individuals want for themselves at the end of their lives should be honored and respected. Mentally capable people who feel that a terminal disease has so destroyed the quality of their lives that they would rather die than go on suffering are entitled to be listened to and respected. Suffering is personal and subjective. How much is bearable is up to the patient and no one else.

Even with advance directives, more people than ever spend their last days in sterile facilities, incoherent, sustained by ineffective pain medications, and tethered to machines that keep them alive but not living. What's worse, these treatments sometimes go against their explicit wishes. According to a study published in the *Journal of the American Medical Association*, "Nearly 40 percent of chronic illness patients nearing their end of life who had physician orders limiting treatment received intensive care that was inconsistent with those orders."[1]

INTENTIONAL DEATH

Dying people ought to be allowed to die peacefully in their sleep with a medication prescribed for that purpose instead of suffering pain, agitation, delirium, air hunger, nausea, and other symptoms, which will only get more severe as time goes on. Terminally ill people should be able to use drugs and other means (such as voluntarily stopping eating and drinking) to access a peaceful death. It's so much better to give people these options than to force suffering individuals to use a gun or another violent means to end their anguish.

An intentional death gives the dying person peace of mind, a sense of agency, the chance to die at home, the end of unnecessary pain and suffering, and reduced trauma for loved ones. A full and meaningful life ending with a sense of completeness and few regrets provides a profound lesson in living and dying well. The family has a chance to gather around the dying person's bedside. Sharing laughter, memories, and healing words can create a sacred and memorable event.

People should be free to shape and design how their lives will be completed when faced with a future riven with pain, suffering, and gross indignities. Episcopal priest and thanatologist John Abraham believes it should be lawful for a competent person suffering unbearably to end life deliberately and intentionally with peace and dignity. He writes, "The right to hasten one's death is the next great civil right" to fight for.[2] He ranks the right to die with dignity (through deliberate life completion) with other ongoing struggles—women's rights, racial rights, disability rights, and LGBTQ+ rights.

"I WOULD RATHER DIE LIKE A DOG"

Causing our own death is not a criminal act and can, under certain circumstances, be a profoundly wise and loving thing to do, especially when one's life is so severely diminished that living is worse than death. If a cherished dog is dying and in pain, the owners ask a vet to end her life painlessly and peacefully. This action is widely viewed as morally decent and merciful. No humane person would let his dog suffer without euthanizing her. Why are humans at the end of life treated worse than dogs?

Advocates for the right to choose death like to use the slogan, "I would rather die like a dog." They mean, "Treat me mercifully, as we treat our beloved pets." My friend Craig Sechler told me, "I continue to be amazed that my English Bull Terrier, Ned, was given a much kinder, nobler death with dignity than was my father, who was under the care of physicians and nurses in hospital."[3]

OPTIONS FOR HASTENING DEATH

The right to determine your own manner and time of death should be universal. The horrors of dementia, cancer, heart failure, and other diseases can lead people to intentionally choose a nonviolent way of dying. What follows is a description of the various ways of hastening death and shortening the period of intense and intractable suffering caused by illness and disease:

- Withholding and withdrawing unwanted life-sustaining treatments
- Voluntarily stopping eating and drinking (VSED)
- Palliative or terminal sedation (what used to be called "barbiturate sedation")
- Lethal medication, including medical aid in dying (MAID)

WITHHOLDING AND WITHDRAWING UNWANTED LIFE-SUSTAINING TREATMENTS

In 1983, Nancy Cruzan was in a car accident that left her brain damaged; she was on life support for the next eight years. She came to represent how cruel intensive medical technology can be and how artificially keeping patients like Cruzan alive is worse than death. Her parents petitioned the US Supreme Court to remove her feeding tubes. In a landmark decision, the court ruled that competent adults have the moral and legal right to refuse any form of medical care. Doing so allows nature to take its natural course.

People facing declining health or dementia who do not want their lives artificially extended can work with their doctors to customize their health-care choices away from extending life. Life-sustaining interventions that can be withheld or withdrawn include treatments and tests, such as mechanical ventilation, intravenous hydration, a feeding tube, cardiopulmonary resuscitation (CPR), and antibiotics. They can be legally declined or stopped at any time, even if they prolong life. This decision can be made by patients or by their health-care agents.

Competent adults (or their health-care agents) can refuse any and all treatment while still being entitled to palliative care to keep them comfortable. There is no guarantee that this will hasten death, but it's likely. Medical providers tend to be hardwired toward testing and treating, so making these sorts of changes will be trickier than it might sound, and one must be firm in pursuing them. If people with dementia decide to permit their dementia to advance beyond the point of their ability to refuse treatment, then they will want to tell their loved ones and doctors, in the dementia provision of their advance directive, to reject or withhold treatment when "the line" is reached.

Voluntarily Stopping Eating and Drinking (VSED)

Voluntarily stopping eating and drinking (VSED), is a practice in which a very ill patient, facing devastating decline, intentionally hastens death by stopping the intake of all food and fluids—that is, refusing food and water (fasting) until death. VSED is available to everyone everywhere (unlike medical aid in dying) and places the dying process in the patient's control. For a person with a terminal condition near the end of life, deciding not to eat and drink is an ethical, legal, effective, and practical way to hasten death. It's a well-understood and socially accepted method of hastening death.

VSED is legally permitted in jurisdictions where medical aid in dying is not. Unlike aid in dying, it's not limited to terminal illnesses or to those with current decision-making capacity. The most authoritative source on VSED is the 2021 book *Voluntarily Stopping Eating and Drinking: A Compassionate, Widely Available Option for Hastening Death*.[4] This book is an invaluable resource for those approaching the end of their lives and seeking guidance and wisdom. It argues that VSED is a caring and compassionate option for accelerating death that respects personal choice. The four authors, all distinguished authorities, say that VSED is typically peaceful when accompanied by adequate palliative care and caregiver support.

Dr. Timothy Quill and his coauthors state, "VSED provides an opportunity to achieve a relatively peaceful, personally controlled death for patients seeking an escape from the prospect of unacceptable suffering or deterioration in their present condition or foreseeable future."[5] Author and end-of-life expert Dr. Sam Harrington says that VSED does not cause significant discomfort and that palliative care can manage symptoms like dry mouth or agitation.[6] He writes, "Any minor hunger pains that occur will be rapidly dissipated by the euphoria of fasting and the sense of taking control."[7] Harrington goes on to say that the sleepiness of dehydration generally replaces this euphoria in a few days. After that, coma and death follow comparatively quietly.

Of course, dying by dehydration and starvation for a healthy person is agonizing and terrifying. But for very ill people near the end of their lives who are resolved to end life on their own terms, the process of dying by VSED is entirely different, provided they work with an experienced doctor, medical team, or hospice. As death approaches, bodily changes often take away the appetite, so VSED aligns with a natural death but should be medically managed to minimize discomfort.

People who choose this option should work with hospice or a medical team. Doctors say that hunger or thirst pains can be minimized for dying people near the end of their lives, especially in hospice care, where narcotics and sedatives can reduce discomfort.[8]

Many people who do not qualify for medical aid in dying may want to consider VSED as an alternative way of hastening their death. For some people, the possibility of using VSED in the future may permit them to continue living fully without the debilitating fear that they will get cornered and trapped with dementia or another horrifying disease and have no means of escape. Unlike aid in dying, a doctor's consent is unnecessary to start VSED, and there are no regulatory hurdles to slow a patient down. It's legally permitted in every state in the United States.

If a mentally competent patient refuses nutrition or hydration, that is his prerogative.

VSED does require grit and determination. Death usually occurs within two weeks, assuming the person diligently avoids drinking. However, death can occur within a few days for someone already weakened. It can be longer than two weeks for those who are strong or take small amounts of liquid. Unlike a chosen death via medical aid in dying, VSED provides a gradual transition for the dying individual and family members. Friends can visit to say goodbye.

Many other societies perceive stopping eating and drinking as a signal that the patient is dying, not as a cause of death. They see inserting a feeding tube in a frail, dying patient as inappropriate. People tend to stop eating and drinking as they approach death, and their organs start faltering and shutting down. As author and hospice chaplain Hank Dunn points out, "It was like we were created to go out of this world as gently as possible, and the way we have done this since the beginning of time is to stop eating and drinking at the end of life."[9]

PHYLLIS SHACTER AND HER HUSBAND, ALAN ALBERTS

Author and teacher Phyllis Shacter was married to Alan Alberts. Alan was diagnosed with Alzheimer's at age seventy-five. He had seen his mother die a horrible and slow death from dementia and did not want to go through that agony or subject his wife to watching him suffer that way. So, in 2013, while he still had the mental capacity to make his own health decisions, he voluntarily stopped eating and drinking to hasten his death.

His wife supported him and wrote a book about the experience called *Choosing to Die*.[10] In her book, Shacter describes how her husband used VSED to gain control over Alzheimer's. He wanted to live as long as he could while mentally alert and capable but did not want to suffer through the late stages of the disease when he would no longer be himself.

Shacter's message is that "VSED is a safe, legal, and comfortable alternative to months or years of suffering and low quality of life."[11] She knows that a person with late-stage Alzheimer's does not recognize loved ones, can behave weirdly, wanders off, gets lost, and may give away precious possessions. Shacter contends, "People who choose to end life voluntarily before having to endure this suffering or put families through it should be permitted to do so."[12]

Alberts decided that VSED was his best option for an elective death, although it raised vexing questions for the couple, questions to which there are no easy answers:

1. What is the best time to initiate VSED?

2. How can you avoid starting too early to prevent the risk of starting too late when cognitive decline makes VSED impossible?

3. How do caregivers respond to the patient's thirst when the patient no longer remembers why he is not drinking?

4. Should hospices help patients who opt for VSED to lessen their suffering?

VSED requires that the person have decision-making capacity (e.g., does not have advanced dementia). What about people who do not want to hasten their death in any way until *after* they lose their decision-making capacity? This is a complex issue, but Dr. Timothy Quill and his coauthors have addressed it comprehensively in their book *Voluntarily Stopping Eating and Drinking*.[13]

In these and all situations, VSED ideally should be supported by hospice, and the dementia must be early enough for the person to be mentally capable of remembering the choice to stop eating and drinking. Individuals should make a video in their most lucid time to use as a reminder of their intentions. Final Exit Network (discussed later in this chapter) is working to provide and legally support an advance directive with which competent individuals can specify that their future incompetent self (when they have advanced dementia) can use VSED to hasten their death.

DIANE REHM AND HER HUSBAND, JOHN REHM

NPR radio host and author Diane Rehm, a champion of the right-to-die movement, believes that dying people should have the right to determine when their lives should end. She writes, "After watching my husband John suffer terribly at the end of his life, I strongly believe in our right to choose when we die if our illness is beyond any hope of meaningful recovery."[14]

Her husband of fifty-five years, John Rehm, was in a situation similar to Alan Alberts's but was devastated by Parkinson's disease rather than Alzheimer's. John Rehm begged his doctor for medication to hasten his death and help him die, but his doctor refused because prescribing such medication was not legal in Maryland, where the Rehms lived. So, John Rehm chose to hasten his death using VSED.

TERMINAL (OR PALLIATIVE) SEDATION

Even strong medication cannot control severe and relentless pain for some patients. If the suffering from pain, nausea, delirium, agitation, shortness of breath, and other end-of-life miseries becomes too intense and overpowering as death approaches, doctors can sedate a patient with medications to make the patient unconscious. In this calm and comatose state, the patient can die peacefully.

Medical providers call this terminal sedation (other names are palliative sedation, total sedation, and continuous deep sedation). Terminal sedation is consistent with the Hippocratic oath to do no harm because it's harmful to patients to allow them to suffer without relief. Doctors administer enough drugs to make patients unconscious until they eventually die of their disease, usually within days. It's best done with the help of hospice care to ensure the patients and their loved ones are as well supported as possible. Legal everywhere, terminal sedation prevents further physical and psychological suffering and can hasten the dying process. Many people consider it a humane option for a peaceful death, and needs to be more widely understood.

I salute the nonprofit organization Compassion & Choices for helping to legitimize terminal sedation as a recognized medical practice. In the US Supreme Court decision, Vacco v. Quill (1997), Compassion & Choices advanced the case that recognized dying patients have a constitutional right to receive as much pain medication as necessary, even if it advances the time of death.[15] The guiding ethical principle at the heart of terminal sedation is that of the "double effect." Terminal sedation is considered ethical as long as doctors are not intentionally trying to hasten death. This legal legerdemain (the doctrine of "double effect") allows physicians to treat patients' pain while knowing it will likely kill them.

The creed or moral principle of "double effect" (first formulated by the Catholic theologian St. Thomas Aquinas in the Middle Ages) holds doctors innocent of murder if they deliver powerful drugs (like opiates) to dying patients to relieve their unbearable pain and suffering, and those drugs, simultaneously and as a side effect, hasten death. An action is judged by its primary purpose or intention. Navigating insidious diseases like Parkinson's, heart disease, cancer, ALS, and emphysema will likely, at the end stages, bring patients and doctors face-to-face with the double-effect doctrine.

TERMINAL SEDATION VERSUS EUTHANASIA

Euthanasia, an illegal and criminal act in the United States, is when a doctor delivers a lethal dose of medication to a patient, usually at the patient's request, with the intent to terminate the patient's life. Terminal sedation is defined similarly, except that the doctor ostensibly gives the lethal dose to ease a patient's agonizing and unrelenting pain and suffering, even though the doctor knows full well that the drugs will make the patient unconscious and bring about death. Palliative care and hospice doctor Shahid Aziz says, "The intention in euthanasia is to hasten death by willfully giving life-ending medicines. On the other hand, in terminal sedation, the intention is to relieve suffering by giving just enough meds to take away the pain and suffering and then letting nature take its course."[16]

There is, in reality, a barely visible difference between euthanasia and terminal sedation. While there is a distinction between a doctor medicating dying patients until they are unconscious to ensure they feel no pain and injecting the same patients with the intent to stop their breathing or their heart, in practice, this distinction is murky. Both shorten life and hasten death, but the second action intentionally ends life. "Terminal sedation," writes cardiologist Dr. Haider Warraich, "bears an eerie similarity to euthanasia."[17] Euthanasia in the United States is intensely controversial, but terminal sedation, which also hastens death, is not. Terminal sedation is practiced by medical providers everywhere and is perfectly legal.

The double-effect ethical principle allows for unintended harm, including a patient's death, if the doctor is well intended and striving toward an obvious good—the relief of suffering. The distinction between letting terminally ill people die and intentionally ending their lives can get opaque. A precept of palliative care is not to deliberately hasten death, but this precept is soft and mushy in practice.

MEDICAL AID IN DYING[18]

Medical aid in dying (MAID) is when a doctor writes a lethal drug prescription for a terminally ill patient who self-administers the drug and dies. It is patient driven, not doctor driven. The patient must have a prognosis of six months or less to live, have decision-making capacity (i.e., be mentally capable), and be able to take the medication himself if and when he decides to. More generally, MAID refers to the legal practice where a clinician cares for terminally ill patients as they consider and potentially follow through with hastening their imminent deaths.[19] In states where aid in dying is authorized and legal, patients can exit life with an intentional, planned death to escape agonizing, relentless deterioration at the end of life.

The widespread use of antibiotics has brought a damaging and unplanned consequence. In the pre-antibiotic era, the duration of prolonged deterioration with extensive suffering before dying was significantly lower. Patients typically would rapidly contract infections, such as pneumonia, which would end their lives. Modern medical technology has forcefully restrained nature's most common way of alleviating protracted suffering. MAID provides a compassionate and humane alternative.

MAID allows terminally ill adults to request and receive a prescription for medication, which they may choose to take themselves—by mouth, by a tube inserted through the skin into the stomach wall,[20] or rectally. After taking the fast-acting drugs, patients fall asleep within a few minutes, drift into a deep coma, and then segue peacefully and painlessly into death.

Those who choose to end their suffering using MAID do so because of loss of autonomy, decreased ability to participate in activities that make life enjoyable, and loss of dignity. Surprisingly, few do it because of physical pain. Often their suffering shows up as exhaustion and fatigue. A patient will say to their doctor, "Doc, I'm so tired. I've had enough." Such patients are ready to exit life and want the autonomy to do that.[21]

Excellent hospice and palliative care can reduce the need for MAID, and that is always to be welcomed. Almost all those who access MAID are on hospice care at home, with hospices that support the use of MAID (not all do). The American Clinicians Academy on Medical Aid in Dying, founded and led by Dr. Lonny Shavelson, has a patient-to-doctor referral service for those seeking a MAID provider; it can be found at www.acamaid.org. Shavelson, one of the leading experts in America on MAID, recommends that an experienced doctor or nurse be with the dying patient when the fatal drugs are self-administered and that the patient have hospice care to ensure strong emotional and clinical support for the patient and family.[22]

STRONG PROTECTIONS ARE NEEDED

Strong protections are built into MAID, but the precise protections vary by state. Typically, the patient must request MAID three times, including once in writing, with two witnesses. In addition, two medical providers must certify that the person meets the eligibility criteria. Such protections are needed because some families try to hasten death for unacceptable and immoral reasons. Perhaps the dying person is exhausting the family's savings, was violent and abusive, or is simply an enervating and excessive burden. Or maybe family members seeks their inheritance, which they can't access while the patient is alive.

We must also not be naive about the other direction in which unethical conduct can take us. For example, families sometimes want to keep loved ones alive and prevent them from having a natural and peaceful death because this helps them avoid dealing with death (and perhaps facing their own mortality). Or, they want to continue receiving financial benefits flowing to the patient, preserve their jobs as caregivers, or continue living in the patient's home. For all these reasons, MAID must be conducted with the utmost care.

CRITICS OF MAID

MAID is a polarizing and fraught issue. Critics of MAID claim that it denies God's will, cuts life short, violates the doctor's pledge to do no harm, promotes suicide, and makes euthanasia more acceptable in society. In traditional Christian and Jewish thought, the body belongs to God, so ending one's life is not considered within the scope of a person's authority. Those opposed to MAID laws, including the Roman Catholic Church, feel that any right to die would naturally devolve into coercive pressure to die on the disabled, enfeebled, senile, and debilitated. There is no evidence that this is happening. While MAID has been in effect in Oregon since 1997, there has never been a credible, documented case of abuse.

There is no evidence of a "slippery slope" in which criteria are relaxed, or patients coerced to participate, and there is no evidence that MAID targets minorities or the disabled. Some palliative-care doctors believe that every form of suffering can be alleviated and, thus, MAID is unnecessary. But the scientific evidence for that claim is thin, as evidenced by the occasional (some doctors think it may be frequent) use of terminal sedation on dying patients.

Eleven US jurisdictions, beginning with Oregon in 1997, and including Washington, DC, currently authorize MAID. The MAID laws in those jurisdictions are among the most restrictive in countries with such laws. That hasn't stopped opposition from some religious and right-to-life groups. The Catholic Church (with Mormons and evangelicals not far behind) has invested large amounts of money and resources to oppose the right to choose one's end of life because of the belief that only God should determine when and how one dies.

Some elements of the disability community, for example, the organization Not Dead Yet, also have opposed MAID.[23] They fear that MAID would enable doctors and families to encourage people with disabilities to shorten their lives for selfish and self-serving reasons.[24] As already noted, since 1997, when MAID became law in Oregon, there have been no instances of abuse of the law. No patients with disabilities have been coerced to accept MAID.

Criticism of MAID also comes from those who think *it does not go far enough* and that, for example, MAID discriminates against people with neurodegenerative diseases and neuromuscular disabilities, such as ALS (amyotrophic lateral sclerosis or Lou Gehrig's disease) and Parkinson's. The fear is that people with disabilities might be unable to access MAID when needed.

Some people who support the right to compassionate options for ending one's life believe MAID should be expanded to cover people with dementia and those who cannot self-administer the prescribed end-of-life drugs. Under MAID, patients must self-administer their medications, but those with physical limitations may not be able to do so at the time they wish. This may be true even though physically assisting a patient with MAID is legally allowed and is not a felony. Family members, nurses, and doctors can hold a cup for a patient, mix the medication, put in the PEG tube, and so on.

SUPPORTERS OF MAID

Many people feel that MAID is a fundamental human right. They believe MAID gives a dying person agency, autonomy, and choices. It offers a path to cease suffering from dependency, pain, existential despair, indignities, or whatever else is causing the dying person to feel distressed and wretched. For many dying people, having the option of ending their lives if they want to is itself a relief. About a third of the patients prescribed fatal drugs never use them,[25] but having them available gives patients a gratifying sense of control and agency over their lives.

Supporters of MAID don't believe it violates the Hippocratic oath to "do no harm." Harm is prolonging intense suffering for terminally ill people at the end of their lives, and MAID is designed to end such suffering. It's rational and wise for patients to choose death rather than experience the misery and degradation that their disease will thrust on them. Respecting patients has as much to do with supporting their dignity, autonomy, and relief of suffering as it does with maximizing the number of days they keep breathing.

Respecting values and choice applies to doctors as well. Enacting MAID should not *require* any doctor to assist in a patient's death. Participating in MAID is optional. Doctors can decline to get involved. However, people should be able to find and access safe, compassionate, competent medical assistance in ending their lives.

MAID IN THE UNITED STATES

With MAID permitted in eleven US jurisdictions, one in five Americans has this legal option today. As welcome as that is, it still means four in five Americans *do not have this choice*. Very few people die by MAID—only about three of every one thousand deaths. For a list of states and jurisdictions where MAID is legal, go to deathwithdignity.org/states.

MAID is covered by most private insurance and Medicaid in several states (California, Hawaii, New Mexico, and Oregon). While some patients have to pay for the fatal drugs out of pocket (and they are expensive), many people are covered.[26]

MAID SUPPORT WITHIN MEDICAL ORGANIZATIONS

As this book was nearing completion in mid-2023, the nonprofit organization Compassion & Choices reported that MAID continues to gain acceptance in health and medical organizations. Over the past six years, thirty national and state medical and professional associations have endorsed MAID or dropped their opposition to it.

Major national organizations, including the American Public Health Association and the American College of Legal Medicine, have adopted support for MAID. At the same time, the American Academy of Family Physicians, the American Academy of Hospice and Palliative Medicine, and the American Nurses Association have dropped their opposition in favor of engaged neutrality toward MAID, respecting their members' varying views while providing accurate information and education.

These changes demonstrate that acceptance of MAID within the medical field is gaining momentum. Independent national and state surveys show that the American public consistently supports MAID by large majorities.

MAID and Brittany Maynard

MAID received a colossal boost in 2014 when Brittany Maynard, a young teacher in California who suffered from a particularly virulent form of brain cancer, made a YouTube video that was watched by millions. Maynard wanted to hasten her death so she and her family would be spared the intense suffering her disease would inflict on her. California did not, at the time, allow MAID, so Maynard and her family moved to Oregon. There she took lethal drugs lawfully prescribed by a doctor and died peacefully.

Brittany Maynard was not choosing between living and dying. Her only choice was between two ways of dying—one gentle and the other filled with pain. She showed that MAID is one of the most selfless gifts dying people can give their families. Her YouTube video and press interviews sparked major support for the right to plan your death and die intentionally. MAID was made legal in California in 2015. Before Brittany Maynard died, she wrote,

> After months of research, my family and I reached a heartbreaking conclusion: There is no treatment that would save my life, and the recommended treatments would have destroyed the time I had left. . . . Even with palliative medications, I could develop potentially morphine-resistant pain and suffer personality changes . . . of virtually any kind. . . . I am not suicidal. . . . I do not want to die. But I am dying. And I want to die on my own terms.[27]

Everyone should have access to MAID as an additional choice alongside palliative care, hospice care, terminal sedation, discontinuing treatments, and VSED.

Amy Bloom and Her Husband, Brian Ameche

For Americans who yearn to end their suffering from painful diseases but cannot access MAID because it is not legal in their state (and who are unwilling to use VSED or a violent method, such as a gun, to end their lives), another option is to go to Switzerland to take advantage of that country's progressive laws. The Swiss approach allows a patient of sound

mind to plan and put into practice a self-determined ending of life and suffering by her own action, accompanied by a nonprofit organization and involving the support of medical doctors. The Swiss believe that mentally qualified people should be able to end their lives in a dignified way consistent with their values and preferences, even if they are more than six months away from dying.

Switzerland allows non-Swiss citizens to visit Switzerland to access MAID. Including travel, this can cost between $10,000 and $20,000. So it's expensive, and the paperwork is onerous. The Swiss nonprofit organizations Dignitas, Pegasos, and Lifecircle can provide information on their criteria and what is needed.[28]

Novelist Amy Bloom's book *In Love: A Memoir of Love and Loss* tells the story of her experience traveling to Switzerland with her husband, Brian Ameche. Brian wanted to "die on his feet rather than live on his knees," so he decided to hasten his death when he was diagnosed with Alzheimer's. Ameche could not find what he wanted in the United States because, in the jurisdictions where MAID is legal, you have to be terminally ill with less than six months to live. So he felt his only option for a painless, peaceful, legal, and self-determined death was in Switzerland.

Medical Aid in Dying Is Not Euthanasia

Euthanasia comes from Greek and means literally "a good death." It refers to a process (illegal in the United States) in which a patient's life is ended by a doctor using lethal drugs, like a veterinarian putting a dog "to sleep." In contrast, with MAID, a doctor writes a lethal prescription for a patient with a terminal disease to end life *by his own hand*. In euthanasia, the doctor or nurse takes the action that hastens death. In MAID, the patient is in charge and has autonomy.

Pathologist Jack Kevorkian popularized euthanasia in the 1990s. He helped dozens of patients die and eventually went to prison for his activities. An argument against euthanasia is that it might devolve into the involuntary killing of the aging and disabled.

Voluntary euthanasia is where a doctor directly injects lethal drugs at the patient's request. This is permitted in several countries, including Canada, the Netherlands, Belgium, and Luxemburg. In Australia, Exit

International's Dr. Philip Nitschke was the first doctor in the world to provide voluntary euthanasia legally.[29]

MAID IS NOT SUICIDE

Opponents of MAID prefer to call it "assisted suicide" or "physician-assisted suicide." Opponents do this because they know that the word "suicide" has pathological, illegal, and even criminal implications for many people and therefore serves to undermine MAID. But an ill person near the end of life who desires a hastened death no longer enjoys the possibility of a worthwhile and meaningful life. It makes little sense to compare a mentally capable, terminally ill person who will die soon from an underlying disease with a mentally troubled person who may be young and healthy and prematurely ends life alone, often violently.

In the Western world, suicide has historically been viewed as shameful. For many centuries, people who committed suicide were considered criminals, and their families were sometimes punished, for example, by confiscation of their property. People who survived suicide attempts were punished with imprisonment. Suicide became decriminalized thanks to the development of science, humanism, the Enlightenment, and the growing separation of church and state. There should be no limits on an individual's right to self-determination and freedom of choice concerning the end of life. It diminishes the pressure on them to resort to violent suicide attempts.

When people die by suicide, they often use violence (i.e., with a rope, a gun or through drowning or suffocation) to take their lives. Violent (and almost always lonely and risky) means of ending life are available but come with horrific side effects, including trauma for the survivors, compared to using drugs with a doctor's legal involvement.

The word "suicide" in our society has a negative and stigmatizing tone for good reasons. It's traumatic, horrifying, messy, and violent, ending the possibility of a worthwhile and meaningful life. MAID is an option for the dying that spares the person (and their family and friends) unbearable suffering and offers a controlled and peaceful ending. Terminally ill patients who seek MAID are not suicidal in the common understanding of that word. Without their illness, they would have no desire to hasten their death. Increasing numbers of people view hastening death using MAID as a thoughtful, rational response to avoid further suffering from severe conditions. A better word than suicide in this context is "self-deliverance."

A suicide typically ends the life of someone expected to live a long time. It is profoundly shocking and devastating to the family of the deceased. In contrast, hastening death at the end of life through MAID gives agency to the patient so she can achieve death with dignity and be surrounded by loved ones.[30] As MAID expert Dr. Lonny Shavelson writes,

> suicide is when a person has the possibility of living on. . . . A person with a terminal illness who qualifies for medical aid in dying, on the other hand, has no possibility of living on. . . . Their choice is how they will soon die, not if they will soon die. They are not rejecting life, and they've often fought as hard as they could to prolong their life by aggressive medical interventions. Now, they are choosing the route to their rapidly approaching death—unwanted but inevitable. That is not suicide. For this reason, all medical-aid-in-dying laws clearly state that medical aid in dying is not a suicide—not for life insurance, not on the death certificate, not for medical records, not for any legal or other document."[31]

Note to readers: If you are having thoughts of suicide, call or text 988 to reach the National Suicide Prevention Lifeline or go to SpeakingOfSuicide.com/resources for a list of additional resources.

WHEN TO INGEST THE MAID MEDICATION

Patients with advanced and incurable neurological diseases may be unable to ingest the MAID medications without major assistance. The fraught legal and moral question is as follows: Should such patients be allowed such assistance, or is that euthanasia and therefore illegal in the United States? Denying assistance in ingestion to a neurologically compromised patient is unlawful because it violates the Americans with Disabilities Act, which says that people with disabilities should have the same rights (and equal access) as the nondisabled.

MAID's insistence on self-administration places the affected patients in an untenable and nightmarish position, forcing them to choose between acting sooner while they are physically able to self-administer the fatal drugs without assistance or waiting and possibly losing the ability to take the medication, then enduring a painful, extended death.

LEONARD LEVENSON'S STORY

In the Fall 2020 Final Exit Network (FEN) newsletter, FEN member Leonard Levenson explained how his mother wasted away over seven years due to Alzheimer's. He wrote that his confirmed genetic profile increases his chances of a similar fate. Levenson has told his family that, when the time comes, he hopes to die peacefully by his own volition and not endure years of abject pain and suffering with no quality of life. At the end of his life, he said he would like to be surrounded by his loved ones and celebrate the extraordinary gift of life itself. They will talk and enjoy the fact that they shared so much. They will say their farewells, and then Levenson will take an appropriate "elixir" that will carry him gently out of existence. He says such an ending would be "a satisfying one to my life's story."

Unfortunately, as already noted, the current US MAID laws require the patient to trigger his own death. But Levenson worries that, with Alzheimer's, he won't have the capacity to do it himself. This means he may be forced to execute a "self-inflicted death" or SID, which he finds appalling. He said, "If my life's quality diminishes to the point where living becomes unacceptable to me while I still possess the mental and physical capacity to kill myself, I will."

In other words, unless the laws are changed to allow for his desired peaceful end, he will be forced to experience a premature, self-administered, possibly violent act, committed alone while angry and afraid. He will become another statistical suicide, leaving his family in pain. He argues that he should not have to resort to a self-inflicted death. No one should have to resort to a gun, a rope, or drowning. Everyone should be able to die surrounded by loved ones and feeling at peace. Levenson believes there is no moral justification for others to deny him the liberty to pursue his desired kind of death. He wants the laws to be changed to allow people to end their lives on their terms, acquire the means to do so, and get help from someone else if they need it.

Current laws deny access to MAID for thousands of suffering Americans, either because they have dementia or because patients with incurable diseases like multiple sclerosis, ALS, and Parkinson's are not terminally ill and are unlikely to die within six months. MAID laws are useless for these two groups.

FINAL EXIT NETWORK (FEN) AND THE RIGHT TO DIE

FEN is a nonprofit organization working to provide choice in dying. FEN's Exit Guide Program has trained volunteers who educate people on how to comfortably and safely end their lives; they sit with them when they do it so they won't be alone. The guides simply provide comfort and diminish isolation and loneliness. They offer information and support to people in their homes and at no charge. They do not provide tangible physical assistance in death and do not provide the means to bring about death. Anyone working with a FEN Exit Guide must be able to procure, assemble, and operate the equipment needed without help.[32]

FEN keeps abreast of research on safe and reliable methods of self-deliverance so that people can choose to end their lives comfortably at home without having to depend on MAID or the medical system. (Self-deliverance means acting on one's own without a physician assisting.) FEN supports the idea that any competent person suffering from an unendurable and intractable medical condition should have the option of a legal, dignified, and peaceful death. A person can qualify for FEN services without necessarily being terminally ill.[33] For example, FEN works with individuals who are in early-stage dementia and are still mentally capable.

FEN's Medical Evaluation Committee, composed of physicians and health-care professionals, carefully screens applicants to FEN's Exit Guide Program. The program does not accept applications based on mental illness. In addition, the committee requires family members to be aware of their loved one's intentions.[34] Operating under the protection of the First Amendment, FEN exit guides provide nothing but information, that is, speech. Thaddeus Pope, a legal expert on end-of-life issues and coauthor of the book *Voluntarily Stopping Eating and Drinking*, says, "Merely advising a patient about how to hasten their death does not constitute 'assisting' a suicide within the meaning of state felony statutes. So, the conduct of FEN exit guides is generally not illegal, though a few states have construed the word 'assist' to cover mere speech."[35]

* * * * *

Arguably, the greatest of our civil liberties is the right to govern our lives, including the right to choose when and how to die. Those patients who intentionally hasten their death deserve understanding, compassion, and even admiration. I'm not recommending that all patients with debilitating terminal illnesses hasten their deaths through VSED, MAID, or other means. But those who choose to go that route should not be condemned. It would be facile and wrong to claim that dying patients who want to hasten their deaths are clinically depressed. Most are just rational and realistic. They know a lingering, painful, inhumane death is best avoided.

This chapter has discussed the fraught issue of the right to choose when and how to die. But what is it like to die? We turn to this question in the next chapter.

CHAPTER 9

What Is It Like to Die?

NO ONE KNOWS WHAT IT'S LIKE TO DIE BECAUSE ANYBODY TALKING about it has never experienced it and can only be guessing when it comes to observing someone else dying.[1] Many of us have questions and worries about what death will be like; some examples follow:

- After I die, will my life have any meaning?
- Will my life have mattered?
- Will anyone miss me when I'm dead?
- Will anyone remember me?
- Will I be on a ventilator and unable to say goodbye to my family?
- Will I be struggling to breathe and experience the panic of air hunger?
- At what point will I realize that it isn't a future self that will die but my present self?
- When will I feel the full force of realizing I will soon cease to exist?
- How long will dying take?
- Will I hate my extreme deterioration and diminishment?
- Will my appearance be repellent and ugly?
- Will I have a lingering death and cause my family to be burdened and exhausted?
- Will I lose control of my bowels and bladder?

- Will I feel embarrassed when a stranger or a loved one has to wipe my bottom and change my diaper?
- Will I lose all dignity and privacy?
- Will I have unfinished projects, like an unfinished legacy letter or memoir, that I desperately want to finish?
- Will dying hurt?
- Will I say or do something embarrassing?
- Will I feel lonely?
- Will I be subject to an autopsy and be horribly mutilated?
- Will decomposition turn my body into something disgusting and gruesome?

It's hard to answer those questions. Moreover, the expected way of death for any patient depends on many variables, including the specific diagnosis (if a disease is present), the disease progression, and which body organs are failing the most quickly.

As noted earlier, 80 to 90 percent of us will die gradually from disease or old age. Only 10 to 20 percent of us will die suddenly from such causes as heart attacks, auto accidents, and suicides.[2] Author and hospice nurse Barbara Karnes says that, when people die slowly, they die, for the most part, in a way that reflects their character and personality and how they've lived.[3]

If you're irritable and grumpy, this is likely what you'll be like as you die. If you are relaxed and easygoing, your death will likely reflect the same characteristics. Dying is just one more experience in life, and you will deal with it in the way you have addressed and faced other life challenges. Barbara Karnes says, "Dying doesn't change us, it intensifies our personalities." If people have been cranky, testy, and obstinate in their regular lives, they will likely be even worse as they approach death.

Type-A personalities who always want to be in control and productive are unlikely to spend years (or even months) lying helplessly in a bed in a nursing home; this would be intolerable and unacceptable to them. On the other hand, someone who's content to spend hours watching television may be okay with spending a year or more in a nursing home, lying in bed with the TV on.

Dying may not be pretty. An implacable and ravaging illness can undermine a patient's sense of who he is. A patient's identity, what gives life purpose and meaning, can wither, which may bring on feelings of profound despair. When deteriorating, patients are no longer those things that once defined them—father or mother, husband or wife, nurturer, initiator, organizer, caregiver, breadwinner, family cheerleader, productive worker. They're no longer living as they did at their peak. The work, projects, and accomplishments that helped to give their life meaning are in the past.

The strong, independent, capable, and loving person a patient once was painfully fades away, and the memories of that person in peak health may grow faint. A dying patient can no longer fulfill responsibilities and has become a burden to others. Sickness and senility leave a dying patient a far less appealing and attractive person. In the face of losing responsibilities, roles, and abilities, is it still possible for a dying patient to have mastery in some sense? How does such a patient avoid feelings of helplessness, loss of dignity, fear, and despair?

Having a Purpose

Karnes believes that having a purpose helps us as we approach the end of our lives.[4] Without that, the will to live may languish and wilt. The purpose can be to spread joy; finish a legacy letter; go through photos with grandchildren, identifying who people are; organize scrapbooks; call friends to say goodbye; do a craft project; record family history; or anything else that helps to give life meaning.

One thing we can do right up to the time we lose consciousness before death is to set an example of how to die with courage, dignity, gratitude, and serenity. Modeling what a good death looks like is a beautiful gift for those witnessing our demise and imbues our life with significance.

When dying loved ones are still aware, engaged, and able to talk in the months and even years before death, it is good to talk about their life and reflect on what it has meant. We can help dying people process and better understand the events they lived through by sharing stories, asking questions, looking at photos, and reminiscing.

WHEN DEATH IS A COUPLE OF MONTHS AWAY

If you are caring for a dying loved one and haven't yet thanked that person for all she has done for you, do it before the opportunity slips away. Talk about happy memories, how much you love her, and how grateful you are that she has been in your life and for all she has done for you. Speak from the heart, open up, and reveal your most loving thoughts.

Be engaged, be empathic, and listen intently if the dying person can speak. Thank the person for what he has meant to you. Express how he has enriched your life. Tell the person that you will pass on the values and stories you learned from him to others and that the person will not be forgotten.

Expressing gratitude to a person is too often done solely in a heartfelt eulogy, but we must express appreciation *before* loved ones die and when they can still hear and understand. Too many of us have wistfully reflected at a funeral or memorial service how we wished the deceased were still alive to hear the tributes. This is the notion behind the "toast" letters described in chapter 5.

THE DYING PROCESS BEGINS

Karnes says three things start to happen two to four months before death that "indicate the dying process has begun."[5] The person's eating habits start to change, the person begins to withdraw from the world around her, and the person begins to sleep more and more.[6] Typically, when people finally stop breathing, they are asleep and nonresponsive.[7]

During the hours to minutes before death, while dying patients will likely not respond when you talk to them, doctors think they might be able to hear. So talk to them gently and lovingly. Stroke their face, hold their hand, and, if possible, sit or lie beside them. Some of the signs of dying can be distressing and upsetting to loved ones witnessing them, so the more informed you can be about what happens as death approaches (and hospice nurses are a godsend when it comes to educating families on this), the less alarmed and traumatized you will be by things like the so-called "death rattle" (explained below). Being traumatized by a frightening death can complicate the grieving process. Dame Cicely Saunders, the founder of hospice, once said, "How people die remains in the memories of those who live on."

Robin Ross, RN, a hospice liaison with Montgomery Hospice and Prince George's Hospice in Montgomery County, Maryland, says there are two phases of dying: pre-active and active. But everyone is different, and everybody dies in his own unique way. The two dying phases are just guideposts and should not be taken literally.

The pre-active phase starts perhaps about two weeks before death, and the active phase of dying might last two or three days. In the pre-active dying phase, the patients might be restless, confused, and agitated. They might pick at their sheet, have a decreased attention span, be sleepy, uncommunicative, socially withdrawn, and difficult to arouse. And, of course, they might have pain from any disease afflicting them.

ACTIVE DYING

In the last few days before death, patients are actively dying. Organs like the heart, lungs, and kidneys start shutting down, breathing becomes uneven and even intermittent, and toes and fingers turn blue. The focus of dying patients turns inward (it's usually too late for "last words"), and they drop into a coma before taking their final breath.

Some dying people slip away from life gently and peacefully, but it can be an ordeal for others. They may even have moments of annoyance, anxiety, confusion, or anger. These signs can usually be eased with appropriate drugs but can still be upsetting for loved ones and friends. It's not the peaceful, loving death they hoped for, but they must accept it for what it is. As already noted, doctors and nurses suspect hearing is the last sense to go, so one should always be careful to talk lovingly even though the patient may look comatose.

Watching someone die, even when it is an expected death, can be scary, and it's easy to panic and call 911. However, that is invariably a mistake if the dying person is older because emergency medical technicians (EMTs) are trained to save lives and attempt CPR, even if it inflicts trauma. Far better to have hospice in the home and call the hospice nurse on duty. As noted in chapter 7, nonprofit hospices are the gold standard and will be available 24/7 by phone. They will also be responsive if you need them to come to the home.

When close to death, the dying patient will likely become incontinent (of both urine and stool), might suffer convulsions (or might lie still), and will probably emit a "death rattle." This is when saliva and spit collect in the back of the throat, making a gurgling sound when the patient breathes in and out. A death rattle is usually not distressing to the patient but is difficult for loved ones and caregivers to hear.

The patient stops speaking and may become comatose. The person's breathing becomes sporadic and uneven until it ceases. If agitation and severe pain persist, the hospice team may suggest terminal or palliative sedation (as described in chapter 8). In the final days or hours of life, the body is shutting down and dying. It's a profound, even sacred, event and an intense emotional experience to be with someone you love as the end of life approaches.

What Caregivers and Family Members Can Do

When someone is dying, it's a hallowed, mysterious time. Everyone present will likely reflect on mortality and impermanence. They are bearing witness to a loved one's death. Few things are more precious and memorable. It's scary for everyone because we all fear the unknown. However, the more we can learn from a hospice nurse or other informed person about what will likely happen and what to expect, the less frightened we'll be.

What you do as a caregiver can play a crucial role in how peaceful the death is. Most hospice nurses will recommend staying with the patient as much as possible. Sitting quietly may not seem like much, but it can comfort a dying person. Watch for pain and treat it, or get it treated.

As people are dying, their biggest concern may be losing their dignity (which is often a euphemism for pooping in their diapers), being a burden on their loved ones, or knowing that everyone (or someone in particular) will be all right and properly cared for after they are gone. Some dying people may not want to die with a loved one in the room. It's perfectly okay to say to a person close to death (who may appear unconscious but still be able to hear you) something like, "Dad, I love you. I'm just going to get a bite to eat. It's fine for you to leave whenever you want to—you have my permission to go." In other words, allow them—give them permission—to die if they want to. Barbara Karnes observes that protective parents tend not to die with their child in the room, even if that child is seventy years old.[8]

If you are empathetic and considerate of others, you will likely know how to communicate effectively with loved ones and friends who are sick and approaching the end of life. You are unlikely to make the following mistakes when talking with dying people: "We are going to beat this disease." Or "Let's just talk about something happy." Or "Don't be so negative." Or "You are going to be fine." Or "I see you are in the bargaining stage." Or "This is a blessing in disguise." Or "I'm sure God has a plan." Or "You should try meditation." Or "This is harder on me than on you."[9] Those are not helpful things to say. Instead, listen more and be patient and kind.

Talk from your heart to dying loved ones. Tell them you love them, that you'll miss them, that all will be okay, and that they'll never be forgotten. Gentle, loving, caring words like these can help people die more peacefully and allow caregivers to feel they have done the best job possible. A simple "I love you," or "You have been the best Dad a son could ever ask for," or "I'm so proud to be your daughter," or "I will never forget you," or "You will always live on in my life," all go to help ease the grief and almost certainly comfort and bring peace to the dying.

Say you are sorry about old misunderstandings if you need to. Recall fond memories and retell favorite jokes and stories. Let there be tears and laughter. Then, both parties—the dying and the surviving—can feel that everything that needed to be said has been said. Remember what Winnie the Pooh observed: "How lucky I am to have something that makes saying goodbye so hard."[10] Gather family and friends around the deathbed if the patient wants it. If appropriate, ask dying persons what they would like for their funeral service.

THE HARSH TRUTH ABOUT A FINAL CONVERSATION

While it's essential to communicate meaningfully with loved ones as they approach the end of life, the difficulty of doing so effectively and lovingly underscores why we should talk to them long before the end. Unfortunately, the harsh truth is those final conversations with people before they die, in which profound and loving thoughts are exchanged, do not happen frequently. Dying people often are mentally diminished and physically compromised, but, more importantly, we're often not in the habit of having intimate conversations. Thus, such conversations will not happen comfortably and naturally.

If we want a good death where we express and receive love and caring, we must invest in a good life in which relationships flourish and loving exchanges are said regularly. Unfortunately, loving feelings at the end of life are not guaranteed unless there is preparation for them. The time to talk with our loved ones is *now*, not at some later point, because a better opportunity may never materialize.

Keeping vigil with someone nearing life's end can be awkward. You can quickly run out of things to say. In addition, the dying person may not have the strength to initiate a conversation. Some family members may even choose not to visit the dying loved one because they fear not knowing what to say or do, and observing dying so closely kindles and ignites their own terror of dying. Or they feel fear *on behalf of the loved one* in watching that person die. End-of-life trainer Michael Williams suggests the following three things you can say to help make the dying experience more meaningful and comfortable for everyone:[11]

First, tell the dying person you love her. We all want to know that we are loved. Second, tell your loved one how much she has meant to you, and share specific examples of how the person touched and impacted your life. Third, reassure your loved one that you will be okay. Dying people, says Williams, worry about those they leave behind. So, let your loved one know you'll be fine.

These three suggestions help to lessen any awkwardness when attending to the dying. Also, the love and reassurance you express to the dying loved one will help alleviate grief. When my mother was slowly dying in a nursing home in the last four years of her life, I found it challenging to engage in conversations with her that went beyond the superficial. While recently reading Jane Brody's book *Guide to the Great Beyond*, I came across an idea I wish I had been aware of while my mother was still alive. Brody suggested making a list of "My Mother's Ten Best Gifts" to me and then reading them aloud to her. We would have cried together, shared stories, and enjoyed richer and deeper conversations. And, of course, the list would continue to provide my family and me with happy memories after she died.

Dying Is So Much More than the Disease

Barbara Karnes points out that dying is much more than a patient's disease. It's about the emotional and collective response from family and friends to the person dying. It requires comfort care, communal guidance, and, usually, not too much medical intervention. Comfort care is comfort management, including skin care, positioning, mouth care, alleviating physical pain, alleviating emotional distress, and knowing when it's okay to stop focusing on food. Communal guidance is support and attention to family and significant others involved with a person who can't be fixed.[12]

Dying is a natural process. All you can do as a caregiver is to say loving things to the dying, keep them comfortable and clean, prevent them from getting bedsores by turning them from side to side every two to four hours, and give them sufficient pain medication, such as morphine, to reduce symptoms like air hunger. Playing their favorite music and massaging their hands and feet with soothing oils can also help if the patients enjoy that.

Food and Water

A caregiver can offer ice chips or sips of water if the dying person is alert. Hospice nurses advise not to attempt to give fluids to an unconscious patient but to keep the mouth moist and comfortable with frequent mouth care. The patient will stop eating and drinking as a natural part of dying. The patient *does not want* food or water.

Barbara Karnes, RN, says force-feeding a dying person (because you mistakenly think the person needs food and hydration) can cause pain and discomfort. Of course offer food and water but in a gentle, noncoercive way. The body is shutting down. Karnes says that dehydration will cause the calcium level in the body to rise, and, when the calcium level gets high enough, the person goes to sleep and doesn't wake up. She says being dehydrated is a gentle and natural way to die.[13]

DEATH ARRIVES

Robin Ross, RN, with Montgomery Hospice and Prince George's Hospice in Montgomery County, Maryland, says that, when a person dies, there's no pulse, no breathing (respiration), and no response to pain stimuli or verbal commands. The eyelids will be slightly open, pupils fixed, jaw relaxed, and mouth open. There will be a loss of sphincter control. As the blood settles, the corpse will gain a waxy pallor.[14]

Sometimes, when death is imminent, it can take days or weeks to arrive. In that lingering time, caregivers can find the seemingly endless wait annoying, vexing, and almost unbearable, even though they love the dying person and may have spent years trying to keep the person alive. All this is normal and understandable.

A cascade of intense emotions may engulf you when a loved one dies. Such feelings might include intense grief, sadness, gratitude, mental fogginess, regrets, and numbness. You might feel dazed, or you might be relieved that the ordeal is finally over.

There are some practical things to attend to soon after death occurs, but, in the meantime, it's perfectly okay to sit with your deceased loved one, if you'd like, and absorb the enormity of what has happened. Let the raw, swirling, gut-wrenching feelings wash over you and soak through you unfiltered, despite the pain and suffering they may bring.

A BRIEF BATHING AND HONORING CEREMONY

Author and science writer Katy Butler points out that washing and anointing the body with oil after death is traditional in many cultures. She describes how nurses are now bringing a beautiful version of this ancient ceremony into hospital rooms.[15] This "bathing and honoring" practice may help loved ones say goodbye. An end-of-life doula could help facilitate it. Only do this ritual or ceremony if it's helpful to you and brings you comfort, solace, and peace.

The ceremony starts with washing and dressing the body (rather than letting the body be taken immediately to a funeral home). A death doula can help with the washing and dressing. Then, the family anoints the body with lavender oil using the following ceremony:

As the hair is anointed with fragrant oil, a family member recites, "We honor her hair that the wind has played with." Next, a dab of oil is gently rubbed on the brow as another family member says, "We honor her brow, the birthplace of her thoughts."

The ceremony continues as follows, with each line said by someone in the room and the deceased's name inserted as appropriate in each succeeding sentence.

We honor your eyes that have looked on us with love and viewed the beauty of the earth.

We honor your nose, the gateway of breath.

We honor your ears that listened to our voices and concerns.

We honor your lips that have shared so much wisdom and knowledge.

We honor your shoulders that have borne burdens and strength.

We honor your heart that has deeply loved us.

We honor your arms that have embraced us and held us.

We honor your hands that have held our hands and done so many things in this life.

We honor your legs that carried you into new places and new challenges.

We honor your feet that forged your path through life.

We give thanks for the gifts you have given us in our lives.

We give thanks for the memories that we created together.

We have been honored to be a part of your life.

MAKING THE DEATH OFFICIAL

At some point, within a few hours of death, someone needs to make the death official by calling a hospice nurse, doctor, or some other medical official, such as a paramedic, who officially pronounces that the person is dead. If the deceased was at home receiving hospice care, the hospice staff will help. Unless you are having a home funeral, you must call a funeral home or mortuary so their employees can pick up the body, but this is not urgent. You can wait a day or two by keeping the body cool with dry ice to slow decomposition.

Having the funeral home arrive quickly and take the body away can be traumatic, so take your time and do this when you're ready. As noted, if you are doing a home funeral, you may not even need a funeral home; more on that follows in the next chapter. You (or someone you delegate the task to) should call family and friends to tell them the sad news.

* * * * *

Once a person has died, the most immediate issue is what to do with the body. That is the subject of the next chapter.

CHAPTER 10

What to Do with the Body

TELLING YOUR FAMILY HOW YOU WANT TO BE TREATED AT THE END OF your life makes good sense, but telling them how you want your body disposed of is trickier. You won't be there, and you want them to do what will bring them peace and comfort. As funeral expert Joshua Slocum, former head of the Funeral Consumers Alliance (FCA), says, they will experience the funeral, but you will not.

Still, the views of the dying person matter, so a balance must be struck between the needs of the living and the needs of the deceased. The way to solve this dilemma, if the wishes of the dying and the wishes of the living conflict, is through reasonable and rational conversation long before death is imminent. Gently inform your family of your preferences and then ask them what would be meaningful, practical, and comfortable for them. This chapter focuses on the numerous ways body disposition can occur. There are more choices than simply conventional burial or flame cremation. (I'm using the term "flame" cremation to distinguish it from "water" cremation.)

FUNERAL PLANNING

Ideally, we should do funeral planning way before we die. Of course, this is unlikely to happen when the death is unexpected, but the sooner we think about our body-disposition preferences, the greater the gift to our surviving loved ones.

Planning a funeral is emotional and costly and must often be accomplished relatively fast. This makes it challenging for those organizing and paying for the event. For some people, planning their funerals before they die is too onerous. A less ambitious (but still commendable) goal would be to have periodic family conversations about funerals (and one's wishes in a general sense).

Such discussions help to introduce the idea that you don't want your family to overspend (if that's how you feel). It also allows everyone in the family to understand what arrangements might cost and introduces your loved ones to the idea that they can do things more hands-on if they are open to that.

You Can Reject the Conventional Funeral Process

You don't have to take the actions most people take when someone dies. It's common for people to call a funeral home, hand over all responsibility to it, and spend little time with the body of the loved one. There is nothing sacrosanct about any of that. You don't have to use a funeral home. You can stay with the body for a considerable time if you want. You can wash and dress the body yourself, although you might find it helpful to get the help of an end-of-life doula, a home funeral guide, or someone who knows about home funerals.

When you're ready, you can take the body yourself to a green burial ground, cemetery, or crematory. The body can be carried in a casket made of cardboard, bamboo, or another inexpensive material. You can draw on the casket and write loving messages on it. You can reject the conventional funeral process and invent an approach more aligned with your values (including environmental values) and those of the loved one who has died.

The Traditional American Funeral

The hallmark of the traditional American funeral in the nineteenth century and earlier was simplicity. A loved one would die. The body would be cared for by family and friends and then carried in a simple wood coffin to the family property, where it would be placed in a hole dug into the earth.

This traditional funeral is what we now call a "green burial." It was not only simple but also inexpensive. Today, we tend to make the mistake of thinking that an expensive and lavish funeral must be chosen to show love and respect for the deceased.

DON'T EQUATE SPENDING ON A FUNERAL WITH LOVE

Don't think that the more you spend, the more respect and love you show for your loved one. The hair on the back of your neck should stand up if a funeral director says things like, "I'm sure you'll want the best for your father," or "Given your position in our community, I'm sure you'll want to select the best package."

The phony connection between respect and money, while beneficial for the bottom line of funeral homes, is ill-conceived and wrong. The best way to show love and care for a loved one who has died is to hold an affordable funeral that is consistent with their values and preferences as well as your own. Many people don't want to waste money on exorbitant and excessive funeral displays.

Today, flame cremation and conventional burial (with embalming, heavy caskets, and concrete burial vaults) are the most common ways of body disposition, but increasing numbers of people realize those two methods are polluting, energy intensive, and wasteful. The Green Burial Council says that conventional burials in the United States go through roughly 77,000 trees, 100,000 tons of steel, 1.5 million tons of concrete, and 4.3 million gallons of carcinogenic embalming fluid yearly.[1] According to the Lancet Commission on the Value of Death, conventional burials are twenty times (and cremations fifteen times) more carbon intensive than some emerging alternatives.[2]

THE HISTORY OF EMBALMING

Historian Drew Gilpin Faust's book *This Republic of Suffering: Death and the American Civil War* describes how embalming first became widely practiced during the Civil War.[3] The families of slain Union soldiers wanted their sons' bodies shipped home by train to be buried on family land. Embalming slowed the decomposition of soldiers killed in battle. It allowed their grieving families to see their lost loved ones in as lifelike a state as possible. In addition, the bodies of soldiers not mangled in combat could appear as if they had died peacefully, making death look like a deep sleep and less frightening. Embalming comforted distraught families during the Civil War era because it restored some elements of what was then seen as a good death. Faust writes, "It offered a way of blurring the boundary between life and death."[4]

Another impetus for embalming came from Abraham Lincoln's assassination on April 14, 1865. His body needed to be transported from Washington, DC, where he died, to his final resting place in Springfield, Illinois. Given the distance and the desire to allow people across the country to pay their respects, it was necessary to preserve Lincoln's body during the two-week journey. Dr. Thomas Holmes, a pioneer in embalming techniques, was tasked with embalming Lincoln's body for transportation. He used a combination of arsenic-based embalming fluids and other preservation techniques to slow down the decomposition process, allowing the body to remain presentable during the long trip.

The public viewing of Lincoln's body as it traveled by train across the country was a significant event in American history. Millions of people lined up along the route to pay their respects to the fallen president. Lincoln's final journey reinforced the practice of embalming as a desirable way to preserve the bodies of loved ones for viewing during mourning and funeral ceremonies. As a result, embalming gained popularity and became more widely accepted in the United States, leading to the emergence of the funeral industry as we know it today.

THE AMERICAN FUNERAL INDUSTRY AND BUYER BEWARE

Any discussion of the current funeral industry must include the pioneering work of investigative journalist and author Jessica Mitford. She came from the English aristocracy and condemned the US funeral industry in her 1963 best-selling book *The American Way of Death*. She bluntly accused "funeral men" of ripping off grieving families. She criticized funeral directors as predators and con artists who took advantage of distraught families by overcharging for funeral and embalming expenses and upselling them on funeral folderol, such as fancy caskets, they did not need.

Mitford's book, which she updated before she died in 1996, is a scathing and mocking denunciation of the funeral industry and global funeral companies such as Service Corporation International (SCI), which she accuses of avarice.[5]

SCI is a significant player in the funeral industry in the United States and internationally. It's one of the largest funeral service providers, operating many funeral homes, crematories, and cemeteries. SCI earns billions of dollars yearly from the thousands of funeral homes and cemeteries it owns. Many were small, family-run, independent businesses that SCI gobbled up. SCI doesn't change the name or look of these formerly family-run funeral homes, so consumers have no idea they are dealing with a multinational conglomerate.

In her book, Mitford vividly describes how the families of John Kennedy and Robert Kennedy got duped and manipulated by Joseph Gawler's Sons Funeral Home in Washington, DC (owned by SCI) into spending far more on the funerals of the assassinated brothers than the families of those slain leaders wanted.[6]

GETTING AMBUSHED AT THE END OF LIFE

You don't buy a refrigerator by walking into a shop that sells them and saying, "I need a fridge. Please tell me which one to buy and how much it will cost." But that's precisely the way we tend to buy funerals. No wonder grieving families, including the Kennedys, get ripped off regularly. We need to shop around, but who can do that when in shock and grieving? We need to think about funeral planning long before dying so we can be intelligent and wise consumers.

Mitford describes how the modern American funeral service provider lies ready to ambush each of us at the end of life. The only way to avoid being manipulated into spending more than needed is to prepare, plan, and get educated. Author and death expert Michael Hebb writes, "The grim reality is that the elderly are taken advantage of for all manner of services, but none so savagely as they are in matters of death and dying."[7]

JESSICA MITFORD'S ACHILLES HEEL

Mitford's influential book encouraged millions to consider flame cremation in a new light. She opted for a minimally fussy, inexpensive flame cremation when she died, and now more Americans choose flame cremation rather than conventional burial. The reason usually given is that cremation is less expensive than a conventional funeral, but another unspoken reason may be that cremation satisfies our desire not to be reminded of our mortality. Cremation annihilates the body and allows us to put this whole death thing behind us and move on. As comedian Jerry Seinfeld observed, "Cremation is like you're trying to cover up a crime. Burn the body. Scatter the ashes around. As far as anyone's concerned this whole thing never happened."[8]

Mitford focused on reducing funeral expenses for the consumer (a worthy goal). What she didn't do, as mortician and author Caitlin Doughty perceptively saw, was change our society's relationship with death. Doughty writes, "It was *death* that the public was being cheated out of by the funeral industry, not money. The realistic interaction with death and the chance to face our own mortality."[9] Mitford's promotion of flame cremation did not help the American public overcome their death-denying tendencies.[10]

The growing demand for flame cremation may reflect society's death phobia. Thomas Lynch, a Michigan poet and a funeral director for fifty years, says, "The stunning increase in cremation is the single greatest change in our funeral practices in our generation or, I'd venture to say, in the last couple of centuries." He adds, "People want the body disappeared, pretty much. I think it reminds us of what we lost." In the United States, Lynch notes, "This is the first generation of our species that tries to deal with death without dealing with the dead."[11]

Jessica Mitford's book, despite its acerbic brilliance, has another flaw, as seen from the present day. Her endorsement of flame cremation sounds off-key and tone-deaf in an era of heightened concern about anthropocentric climate disruption.

THE FUNERAL CONSUMERS ALLIANCE (FCA) AND SHOPPING AROUND

Just before Mitford died, she concluded that little had changed since the first edition of her book was published thirty-three years earlier. Funeral directors were still taking advantage of grieving people and getting them to spend more than necessary. And we know this is still true today because of the excellent work of the FCA and its state affiliates.

FCA is the "Consumer Reports of Funerals."[12] It is a nonprofit organization that aims to educate and advocate for consumers' rights and choices in the funeral industry. It supports fair practices, a wide range of body-disposition options, and finding ways to make a meaningful and dignified funeral affordable. FCA encourages people to seek simplicity if that is what they want. It gently discourages ostentation, wasteful spending, energy waste, and pollution, assuming that's what the family desires. Not everyone wants a simple funeral, and people have the right to do whatever they want. But FCA believes that simple funerals can be dignified and wants to give families the knowledge to plan one in the face of pressure from the funeral industry and prevailing cultural trends.

FCA has local affiliates across the country. The one in Maryland, where I live, is the Funeral Consumers Alliance of Maryland and Environs (FCAME).[13,14] The FCA affiliates are nonsectarian, nonprofit, educational organizations. They were started in the late 1930s (known then as memorial societies) because of the increasing cost of funerals due to the use of embalming and more elaborate, manufactured caskets.

Local FCA affiliates in almost every state aim to preserve, protect, and defend consumer rights in finding meaningful, dignified, and affordable final arrangements. In addition, these local FCA affiliates provide a wealth of unbiased information. They do this through their websites, printed materials, and a public speakers bureau for community gatherings, such as those of clubs, civic organizations, and councils on aging.

Before you die, it's worth your time to visit a few funeral homes (also called mortuaries), talk to the director, assess your level of comfort with them, and do some preplanning. In other words, shop around. Ask neighbors for recommendations, and search the Internet for funeral homes in your area. Comparison shopping is the most effective way to control your funeral spending. Prices vary among funeral homes by as much as 400 percent, even within your city or county. Thousands of dollars are at stake for grieving families. Josh Slocum, the former executive director of the FCA, recommends getting prices from at least five funeral homes. Local FCA affiliates have done cost comparison price surveys that can help.

MEANINGFUL AND AFFORDABLE FUNERALS

Joshua Slocum says that comparing prices for funerals ahead of time can save you headaches and thousands of dollars. In 2011, Slocum and the late Lisa Carlson (the executive director of the Funeral Ethics Organization) authored *Final Rights: Reclaiming the American Way of Death*. It's a worthy successor to Jessica Mitford's book *The American Way of Death*.[15]

Funeral directors may not be the best people to provide a meaningful death ritual because they want the buyer to spend as much money as possible. On the other hand, empathetic and honest funeral-home directors (yes, they do exist) can be godsends because they know so much about the most effective way to dispose of a body in a memorable and appropriate process that aligns with the buyer's values and preferences.

The funeral industry and cemeteries should offer fair prices, post their prices online, provide a wide range of options, never manipulate grieving families for profit, display low-cost caskets instead of hiding them, and encourage (or at least not obstruct) home funerals. In sum, they should comply with or exceed the Funeral Trade Commission's (FTC's) Funeral Rule (more on the Funeral Rule below).

One hundred fifty years ago, funerals happened in homes and were managed by the family. Home funerals with set rituals were routine. Today, people are unfamiliar with the reality of death because it tends to happen in hospitals or nursing homes rather than at home. (Although, recently, there has been an increase in home deaths because of the increased use of hospice.) This lack of familiarity means that people are often scared and upset by death, making shopping for a funeral even more vexing and arduous.

THE THREE MOST COMMON OPTIONS OFFERED BY FUNERAL HOMES

Funeral homes collect information needed to issue a death certificate, embalm the body (if desired), hold a viewing of the body (if desired), and may even perform funeral services (if desired). Three standard funeral arrangements are direct flame cremation, direct and immediate burial, and a full-service (or conventional) funeral where the body is embalmed.

1. *Direct flame cremation* includes picking up the body, filing paperwork, performing cremation, and returning the cremated remains to the family in a plain utility container. There is no embalming or casket and no ceremony.

2. *Direct and immediate burial* includes picking up the body, washing and dressing, placing it in the casket, filing paperwork, and transporting it to the cemetery. There is no embalming, viewing, or ceremony. (The casket is often, but not always, extra.) Some funeral homes include a graveside service. Direct-and-immediate burial costs are charged by the funeral home and do not include the cemetery fees, which can be significant.

3. *Full-service conventional funeral* (often mistakenly called "traditional") includes cleaning, disinfecting, embalming, providing a casket, public viewing, flowers, music, food, a burial plot, funeral and graveside ceremony, opening and closing of the grave, grave liner or burial vault, and headstone.

The prices for each of the three options vary significantly, and this price variation explains why it's so important to comparison shop. But the above three funeral arrangements are not the only ones available, and greener alternatives are now being offered, giving the consumer more options and choices. More on these options can be found below.

DON'T PREPAY FOR A FUNERAL

While the FCA recommends funeral *planning* ahead of time, it advises against *prepaying*. Prepaying is usually unwise because you might change your mind, better funeral alternatives might become available, you may want to use a different funeral home, you may end up dying far away from the funeral home you prepaid, the money may be lost or mismanaged, family members may lose the paperwork, or the funeral home may go out of business. Prepaying does make sense when spending down to qualify for Medicaid or when death is expected.

Regarding cemeteries, a persistent myth is that buying a gravesite in advance means no cemetery costs. This is not true. A grieving family can expect significant fees for opening and closing the grave, a vault, a plaque, and an upright headstone.[16]

THE FTC'S FUNERAL RULE

Author Jessica Mitford lambasted the FTC for its less-than-stellar performance in protecting consumers with the so-called Funeral Rule, which was promulgated in 1984. The Funeral Rule attempted and largely failed to protect the public from the excesses of the funeral industry. Most funeral homes are not fraudulent or dishonest. Still, they all want to make money, and a stressed and grieving family is vulnerable to a persuasive funeral director.

The Funeral Rule gives consumers important rights when making funeral arrangements. For example, the rule requires funeral homes to provide consumers with itemized price lists at the start of any in-person discussions of funeral arrangements, caskets, or outer burial containers. It also requires funeral homes to provide price information by telephone on request. It prohibits funeral homes from requiring consumers to buy any item, such as a casket, in order to obtain any other funeral good or service.

The Funeral Rule also allows you to bring a casket bought from a third party without a handling fee. Unfortunately, some funeral homes will lower the cost of their caskets to remain competitive with third-party caskets but then increase their service fees to compensate. There is one fee that customers cannot decline, and that is the "basic services of funeral director and staff." So, to get the best value and achieve cost savings, consumers should compare prices on both caskets *and* services.

Caskets vary widely from a few hundred dollars for a simple bamboo or pine box to $20,000 and more for a lavish model. If you decide to buy a casket from the funeral home, the director may try to "upsell" you and persuade you to buy a costlier casket, such as a plush model made of rare wood, unnecessary steel, and fancy velvet lining. You should select a casket that aligns with your values.

FUNERAL HOMES SHOULD POST THEIR PRICES ONLINE

The Funeral Rule was crafted before the Internet age, so the requirement to provide price lists only applies in person or over the phone. Today, it's hard to see why anyone should have to visit or call multiple funeral homes to compare prices.

On June 29, 2022, the FCA and the Consumer Federation of America (CFA) released a shocking report that only 18 percent of funeral homes in the United States show customers their prices online.[17] As I write this (June 2023), to increase price competition, the FTC is considering updating its Funeral Rule to direct funeral homes to post their prices online or, if the funeral home doesn't have a website, to make the prices available digitally (and by email).

HOW EMBALMING IS DONE

The embalmer's equipment consists of "scalpels, scissors, augers, trocars, forceps, clamps, needles, pumps, tubes, bowls, and basins."[18] The body is "sprayed, sliced, pierced, pickled, trussed, trimmed, creamed, waxed, painted, rouged, and neatly dressed."[19] In *Smoke Gets in Your Eyes & Other Lessons from the Crematory*, mortician and author Caitlin Doughty graphically describes how embalming is done. First, the blood is removed by making an incision with a scalpel near the throat, then slicing open the carotid artery and pumping a blend of formaldehyde and alcohol through the circulatory system.

Doughty writes, "Perhaps the dirtiest secret about the process of modern embalming is the occult use of a skinny, light saber-sized piece of metal known as the trocar." The pointed tip of the long, silver trocar is "stabbed" into the stomach so that "any fluids, gas, and waste in the body cavity" can be sucked out. The extracted noxious fluid splashes down the drain and into the sewers. Then the trocar reverses direction, and the embalmer pumps a poison cocktail into the chest cavity and stomach. Embalming takes two to three hours to complete.[20] The National Cancer Institute found that embalmers experience higher cancer rates because of their close association with the toxic chemicals in embalming fluid.[21]

Doughty points out that although embalming is not required by law, it's the process around which the funeral industry has evolved over the last 150 years.[22] The funeral industry saw embalming as the key to elevating its social status and having "funeral men" respected as professionals rather than disdained as factotums and body disposers. Embalmers skillfully promoted the dubious story that they created handsome, hygienic corpses to comfort the grieving and protect the living from disease. They portrayed themselves as almost medical and, therefore, deserving generous compensation.[23]

What Embalming Accomplishes

Embalming delays decomposition so that a funeral can be held several days after the death, and cosmetology (more on cosmetology below) restores a lifelike appearance as though the person is sleeping rather than dead. The economic base of the funeral industry, embalming is practiced widely in the United States, yet, outside America, it's viewed as a bizarre social custom and in poor taste. Gazing at the prettified corpse of a loved one, gussied up with makeup, eye caps, and formaldehyde to look like a living doll, is typically seen by non-Americans as a little nutty. Many object to embalming for religious or economic reasons, while others consider it a wasteful and disgusting practice.

Nurse and author Sallie Tisdale describes how shocked she was when she saw her mother's embalmed body because her mother, after a long, debilitating illness, looked "alive again."[24] But Tisdale didn't want that. She didn't want this "false life." She writes, "To this day, I resent what was done to my mother." When we view an open casket, the face of the person who has died is reworked and altered to hide the physical effects of dying.

Does viewing a restored and embalmed body help people through their grief? For some African American communities, the religious and cathartic impact of viewing the body is profound, and embalming plays a positive role in the grieving process. So, for some people, embalming may be important, but I can find little evidence to support the view that seeing an embalmed body is therapeutic for most grieving people. The funeral industry claims that making the deceased look like a living, sleeping person honors the person and preserves good memories of them. That may be true for some, but, for others, it is just as likely to mess with our acceptance of death.

ALTERNATIVES TO EMBALMING

A few decades ago, funeral homes took it for granted that a dead person would be embalmed and would not even ask the family for permission. They would give the impression to grieving families that embalming was a legal requirement (it is not), thus collecting a nice sum of money from the bereaved. Today, more and more people are opting out of getting embalmed. No federal or state law mandates embalming. Some funeral homes ask that a body be embalmed if it is to be viewed, but this is not required by law. Grieving families should ask the funeral home if they offer viewing without embalming and if they can refrigerate the body, which serves, like embalming, to slow decomposition.

It's possible to have an open casket for a viewing without embalming, but the funeral home might say you have to carry out the funeral quickly before decomposition sets in. Refrigeration, like embalming, slows decomposition, but refrigeration is cheaper, less toxic, and less polluting. The chemicals involved in embalming, such as formaldehyde, are highly poisonous and buried with the body and thus may leak into the surrounding area.

A funeral home makes money from embalming and has a vested interest in hoping you will request it. Some funeral homes may not even install refrigeration facilities to avoid having to offer that less-expensive option. If you choose a simple, relatively quick, and straightforward body-disposition method, such as immediate burial or direct cremation, the issues of body preservation and slowing decomposition become irrelevant.

"SETTING THE FEATURES" OR "PREPARATION"

Not to be confused with embalming is something funeral directors call "setting the features" or "preparation." This does not involve preservation but only prettification and cosmetology. Death does weird things to the human face. Caitlin Doughty goes so far as to say that "a dead person's face looks horrific."[25] This doesn't matter except that loved ones like to take one last look at Grandpa before he is buried or cremated, and funeral directors don't want their customers to be horrified. The eyes are open, flat, milky, and sunken. The mouth spreads wide open. The skin is pallid and cadaverous. To correct all these defects, the funeral home will charge several hundred dollars to "set the features" to make the dead person look "natural."

We know what this process involves, thanks to Doughty. "Eye caps" with tiny spikes are placed under the eyelids to keep the eyes closed and rounded. A "needle injector" is then used as a mouth-closing gun that shoots thick wires into the dead person's gums to be tied together to hold the mouth shut. If either of these methods fails to fix the appearance of the eyes or the mouth, then superglue is used to do the job.[26]

The president of the Funeral Consumers Alliance of Maryland and Environs (FCAME), Barbara Blaylock, says,

> Some may find it discomforting to have the facial features set with eye cups and sutured shut eyelids and jaw. Indeed, the results may not look like the actual live person, but many people would probably find it horrifying to see an open gaping mouth and sunken eyes. However, unlike embalming, there is no environmental cost to that bit of cosmetology. Most funeral directors sincerely believe that setting the features is doing the family a great kindness, although they do charge for it.[27]

The funeral cosmetologist also spray-paints the face with makeup and styles the hair, often from a family-supplied photo of the loved one. The funeral home may ask for a dead woman's lipstick to ensure it's the right shade. Older-style funeral homes may still use theatrical pancake makeup, but the air-brushed foundation is the more modern way that makeup is applied.[28]

GRAVE LINERS AND BURIAL VAULTS

Grave liners and burial vaults are another component of conventional burials. They are outer burial containers to hold buried caskets. A grave liner is a concrete encasement that covers and encloses a casket or coffin. It prevents the casket from coming in contact with the earth.[29] Some grave liners do not have a bottom. Thus, both the casket and the grave liner rest on the soil.

Burial vaults, like grave liners, are concrete encasements for caskets. A burial vault contains an inner layer of plastic that is sealed when the body is buried. It does not allow anything to go in or out after it has been sealed. Grave liners and burial vaults are outer receptacles to protect the body and the casket from the depredations of the soil so that the deceased is ostensibly preserved. But liners and vaults will not stop the body from decomposing. Indeed, nothing will.

While no law in any state requires grave liners or burial vaults, many cemeteries require them because they prevent the sinking of the grave due to the eventual disintegration of the casket. Cemeteries dislike bumpy and collapsed ground because it makes mowing difficult, so they may insist on using grave liners and burial vaults even though they are expensive and wasteful.

FLAME CREMATION

In her 1998 book, Jessica Mitford reported that funeral homes and cemeteries have now taken cremation—a low-cost, simple goodbye—and "upgraded it" to extract more money from bereaved families. They raised prices and sell fancy niches and urns to hold cremated remains.

Flame cremation is what most people think of when they hear the word "cremation." It reduces the body to cremated remains or ashes (primarily bone fragments) using the intense heat from flames. The temperature reaches well over 1,600°F (usually involving gas heat). Over half of all Americans opt for flame cremation (rather than burial) as their preferred method of disposition. It's less expensive than conventional burials and is mistakenly thought by many to be more environmentally friendly.

In 2020, 56 percent of Americans who died were flame cremated, more than double the figure of 27 percent two decades earlier, according to the Cremation Association of North America (CANA). By 2040, four out of five Americans are projected to choose flame cremation over conventional burial, according to CANA and the National Funeral Directors Association (NFDA). However, from an environmental perspective, the growth in flame cremation is highly undesirable.

The flame-cremation process comes with environmental burdens and a large carbon footprint. The process releases gases into the open air through an exhaust system, including vaporized mercury from dental fillings. Flame cremating a body uses as much energy as a 500-mile car trip[30] and releases some 250 pounds of carbon dioxide into the atmosphere, roughly the same amount an average American home produces weekly.[31]

The environmental effects of crematoria, categorized as incinerators along with municipal waste and hazardous waste incinerators, are little understood. However, author Sallie Tisdale reports that a few limited surveys in England showed increased birth defects and stillbirths near crematoria.[32]

IMPROVING BODY DISPOSITION

Conventional burials, embalming, and flame cremation are highly polluting and have damaging carbon footprints. With eight billion people on the planet right now, all of whom will die, we need to generate better alternatives for body disposition.

Three methods have emerged as better for the environment than flame cremation and conventional burial: *alkaline hydrolysis* (water cremation), *natural organic reduction (NOR)* (human composting), and *green burial* (natural earth burial).

As author and mortician Caitlin Doughty has said, the American funeral industry has promoted the idea that a dead body should be embalmed, placed in a fancy casket, and lowered into a heavy concrete vault six feet down.[33] This idea treats the dead as something to be preserved and protected. Advocates for Alkaline hydrolysis, NOR, and green burial reject this premise and argue that a dead body should be returned to nature.[34]

ALKALINE HYDROLYSIS (WATER CREMATION)

Bishop Desmond Tutu, a Nobel laureate, an antiapartheid leader, and a long-time advocate for climate protection and MAID laws, asked that his body be disposed of by alkaline hydrolysis because he viewed it as environmentally responsible. Alkaline hydrolysis is more ecologically friendly than flame cremation. It's a quiet, water-based process that reduces bodies to a fine powder, mostly bone material. It is also called water cremation, aquamation, resomation, or biocremation.[35]

During alkaline hydrolysis, a body is sealed in a long, stainless-steel chamber. Three hundred gallons of liquid—a heated solution of 95 percent water and 5 percent alkali (lye or sodium hydroxide)—pass around it. In low-temperature alkaline hydrolysis, the solution reaches a temperature just below boiling, the process is performed at atmospheric pressure, and the body is reduced in fourteen to sixteen hours. In a higher-temperature version of the process, where the mixture tops 300°F and creates more pressure, the body is reduced in four to six hours.

All that's left are a brittle skeleton and a sterile liquid (a combination of amino acids, peptides, salts, sugars, and soaps) safe enough to be discharged into a municipal waste system.[36] The bones are then ground to a fine powder (as in flame cremation) and returned to the loved one's family.[37] Alkaline hydrolysis typically costs under $7,000.

HUMAN COMPOSTING OR NATURAL ORGANIC REDUCTION (NOR)

Human composting (natural organic reduction or NOR) turns human remains into soil (or, more accurately, humus or decomposed organic matter) through microbial decomposition. NOR was first legalized in Washington state in 2019. It's like regular composting, except it's entirely dignified. The body is *not* tossed into a bin with orange peels and banana skins. Recompose, a facility in Washington state, surrounds the dead body with alfalfa, wood chips, and straw in stainless-steel capsules and periodically rotates them at temperatures that naturally rise to 160°F without using energy for heat. That is hot enough to kill almost all disease pathogens and parasites.

After a couple of months, the result is a nutrient-rich, earthy material akin to a cubic yard of fertile soil. This soil can be placed in a grave, scattered in a cemetery, used on trees and plants, or donated to conservation projects. The NOR process not only provides a sustainable and environmentally friendly alternative to conventional burial or flame cremation but also allows the individual to contribute to creating new life. The dead can become nutrient-rich soil used to plant trees and regrow forests.

The long composting period requires maintenance, and the equipment is expensive, so NOR isn't cheap. It costs about $7,000. Medical implants are hand-sifted out and recycled. The soil is also tested for harmful chemicals such as lead, mercury, arsenic, and fecal coliform. During composting, pharmaceuticals, antibiotics, chemotherapy drugs, and other toxins in the body's tissues are reduced to safe levels.[38]

Human composting owes much of its present form to Katrina Spade, a Washington-based urban planner and entrepreneur who founded Recompose and is its CEO. Her goal is for NOR to overtake flame cremation as the default American death care in the next couple of decades.[39] As of mid-2023, seven states—Washington, Oregon, Vermont, Colorado, California, New York, and Nevada—have either legalized or set a date for legalizing human composting as a means of disposition after death. In addition, legislation is pending in several other states. Recompose plans to expand to ten facilities during the next decade. Polls show high interest in green funeral options, including human composting.[40]

Some Catholics tend to oppose NOR. The California Catholic Conference said in a statement, "The methods involved reduce the human body to a disposable commodity, and we should instead seek options that uphold respect for both our natural world and the dignity of the deceased person." However, not all Catholics agree, including scholars who believe Catholics are morally obligated to follow green practices.[41]

GREEN BURIAL

The optimal option for protecting the environment and minimizing carbon emissions is a simple, green burial, the way we have disposed of bodies for eons. A green burial entails returning the body, which has not been subjected to embalming or other processes, to the earth in a setting that does not burden the environment with chemicals or any material expenditure of fossil fuels. The Green Burial Council defines green or natural earth burial as burying "without impediment" to natural decomposition: no embalming, plastic liners, concrete vaults, metal handles, or exotic-wood caskets.

The ideal setting is a dedicated green burial ground or the green burial section of a conventional cemetery. This is a respectful and dignified way to honor the end of life and limit our environmental impact. In addition, it allows the body to decompose and return its nutrients to the earth naturally. Many people want their deaths to reflect their values in life, including respect, appreciation, and reverence for the natural world. Unfortunately, as we have seen, conventional burials, embalming, and flame cremation all violate that wish.

The poet and writer Donelle Dreese says, "These days, when I walk through a cemetery, the kind similar to the one that haunted the landscape of my childhood, I think of formaldehyde, concrete, endless mowing, plastic flowers, glossy caskets, and headstones lined up like gray envelopes in a filing cabinet . . . A walk through a conventional cemetery today leaves me cold and conflicted."[42]

Green burial allows us to escape that conflict and discomfort. At its simplest, green (or natural) burial is the burial of an unembalmed body in a biodegradable container without any burial vault. By its very nature, green burial encourages family and friends to be more engaged in the end of life of a loved one, compared to other more conventional options.

It is a safe and legal way of caring for the dead that embraces the biological processes of decomposition. Green burials have little environmental impact because the body decomposes naturally, often in the top few feet of soil, in biodegradable containers or fabric shrouds, and without embalming chemicals that can leach out. It allows us to face death head-on and choose for our bodies to decompose naturally like those of all other animals.

Dr. Basil Eldadah, who founded and directs the natural burial ground Reflection Park in Silver Spring, Maryland, points out that being culturally sensitive is important. For example, he says, "Some African-Americans shun green burial because it is triggering, as it is reminiscent of earlier days when the bodies of enslaved individuals were disrespectfully buried in the ground without any dignifying accommodations."

LEVELS OF GREEN BURIAL

There are three levels of green burial: hybrid cemeteries, natural burial parks, and conservation burial grounds.

1. *Hybrid Cemeteries* are traditional cemeteries that have set aside a specific portion of their grounds for green burials. Green burial practices are followed in these designated sections, meaning there are no burial vaults or chemical embalming of the deceased. Instead, bodies are interred in biodegradable containers, such as wicker baskets or simple shrouds made from natural fibers. Incorporating green burial areas within conventional cemeteries allows people to choose more environmentally friendly burial practices while still accessing the familiar setting and amenities provided by conventional cemeteries.

2. *Natural Burial Parks* are entirely dedicated to green burials. Natural burial parks are often designed to blend with the natural landscape, embracing the principles of sustainability and environmental preservation. These parks prohibit burial vaults, chemical embalming, and nonbiodegradable caskets or coffins. Instead, bodies are laid to rest directly in the earth using biodegradable materials so that they can return to the soil naturally over time. Many natural burial parks also emphasize the use of native plants and avoid the use of traditional headstones, opting for more eco-friendly markers or tree plantings to memorialize the deceased.

3. *Conservation Burial Grounds* represent the highest environmental responsibility in green burial practices. These grounds are expressly set aside and managed to preserve and protect the natural environment in perpetuity. Conservation easements or legally binding agreements are often implemented to ensure the land remains undisturbed and dedicated to conservation efforts. Burials in these grounds follow the principles of natural burial, with biodegradable containers and no embalming or vaults. By choosing conservation burial, individuals not only reduce their environmental impact but also contribute to the preservation of ecologically significant land areas.

Overall, green burial practices, regardless of the level, prioritize environmental sustainability, ecological consciousness, and a deeper connection with nature. These options provide individuals and their families with choices that align with their values, allowing them to leave a positive impact on the environment even after their death. People who choose conservation burial can die knowing that one of their legacies to their survivors and future generations is protected wild and undeveloped land.[43] In appendix IV, I describe my personal wishes for a green funeral in a letter to my family.

HOME FUNERALS (COMMUNITY-LED DEATH CARE)

Home funerals, which allow families (or communities) to care for their deceased loved ones at home, were common in the United States until the 1930s. The home funeral movement seeks to return to this practice, enabling family and friends to retain custody and control of the body from death until final disposition (burial or cremation). It is a movement to regain the lost skills and self-reliance of our forebears and is driven by a vision of creating more meaningful ways of honoring and caring for our dead.

Sometimes called "community-led death care," home funerals may include the following:

1. Bathing and dressing the body;

2. Sheltering the body at home;

3. Spending time with the body (sometimes called a wake, vigil, or viewing);

4. Filing the death certificate and obtaining a burial/transit permit;

5. Making arrangements for final disposition;

6. Transporting the body for care and viewing and to the place of final disposition; and

7. Making arrangements for any ceremony.

Community-directed death care is legal everywhere in the United States (and the world). For example, in New Hampshire, thanks to activist Lee Webster's leadership, no one is required to purchase the services of a funeral director or funeral home.

"BACK TO THE FUTURE"[44]

In the context of burial practices, "back to the future" refers to a trend in which modern societies revisit and adopt traditional or ancient burial customs. The term highlights the idea that, despite technological advancements and the elaborate funeral industry that emerged in the twentieth century, there is a growing interest in embracing the simplicity and intimacy of older burial practices while incorporating modern values and sensibilities.

In the nineteenth century, home funerals were a common occurrence. When someone died, family members and the local community would gather at the deceased person's home to prepare the body, hold a wake, and conduct the funeral service before burial. This practice allowed for a more personal and involved approach to death care. However, with the rise of funeral homes and embalming in the twentieth century, the practice of home funerals declined. Funeral services became more standardized, and many aspects of death care were outsourced to professionals.

Now, in the twenty-first century, there has been a noticeable resurgence in interest in home funerals and alternative burial practices. Many seek a more eco-friendly, intimate, and meaningful way to say goodbye to their loved ones. The revival of home funerals and the growing interest in greener burial options have been driven by various factors, including environmental concerns, a desire for personalized and authentic experiences, and a general reevaluation of the funeral industry's practices.

BLENDED FUNERALS

Some grieving families select a blended funeral that combines conventional and home funeral practices. A funeral director will take care of certain tasks, such as completing and filing paperwork for the death certificate (which can be onerous) or transporting the body. Blended funerals can be helpful to grieving families who are not familiar with death and dying. Handling a body isn't easy, and a body can be messy when moved (e.g., discharges from both ends of the body are common).

DEATH AND DYING USED TO BE A FAMILY AND COMMUNITY AFFAIR

How people die has changed significantly over the last one hundred years. At the start of the twentieth century, families and communities were familiar with death and dying. They had skills, knowledge, rituals, and traditions related to the end of life that they could apply. Now, death comes later in life for most of us, and ill health and dying last longer. To many of us, death and dying have become unfamiliar. We have outsourced the job to professionals (like doctors and funeral directors) and allowed them to do the work for us.

In the process, we've lost something. The body of a loved one can be lovingly cared for by family and friends, gently washed, then dressed and laid out. This is how it once was before funeral homes became the norm and we hired professionals. Many religious groups, such as Jews, Muslims, and Native Americans, still practice this.

Guests can be invited to say goodbye, and all can, in their own way, dwell on the profound, shocking, and likely devastating event that has just happened—someone deeply loved has died and will no longer be around to interact with physically. Ruminating on the immensity of the life of the person who has just died while spending time with the body can help people absorb the loss and fully grieve.

THE NATIONAL HOME FUNERAL ALLIANCE (NHFA)

It's perfectly legal not to use a funeral home but instead have a home funeral where the body is bathed, dressed, and cared for in the home, followed by a funeral service in the home. There is something mystical and precious about doing this work ourselves with our own hands. Using our own resources in this way and creating our own rituals can effectively ease the pain of sorrow.

Learning to care for one's own dead can be challenging, but there are people who can help. The nonprofit organization National Home Funeral Alliance (NHFA) is an excellent resource for finding local home funeral guides.[45] NHFA educates individuals, families, and communities about caring for their dead.[46]

DISTINGUISHING BEFORE- AND AFTER-DEATH HELPERS

It's essential to distinguish between before- and after-death helpers, their legal scope, and their titles. NHFA supports home funeral guides and after-death care educators, whereas the International End-of-Life Doula Association (INELDA)[47] and the National End-of-Life Doula Alliance (NEDA)[48] train end-of-life doulas who assist *before* death arrives.

Death and dying expert Lee Webster says that "death doula" is a confusing and misleading term we would be better off not using. Better terms are end-of-life doulas (for helpers *before* death) and home funeral guides (for helpers *after* death). Webster has a free video on the distinction between after-death care and care by end-of-life doulas.[49] Home funeral guides who help families with after-death care must be careful not to break any funeral laws or regulations, hospice policies, or cemetery regulations.[50]

FAMILIES' RIGHT TO CARE FOR THEIR OWN DEAD

The home funeral movement, closely tied to the growing interest in green burials and using end-of-life doulas and home funeral guides, is reclaiming the traditional rights of families to care for their own dead, once the standard practice in America. Home funerals give consumers an inexpensive way to circumvent dealing with the funeral industry with its propensity for emotional manipulation and economic deception that cost grieving families unnecessary and significant expense.

Consumer advocate and funeral expert Joshua Slocum writes, "There is nothing the least bit bizarre about families wanting to say goodbye to loved ones in a more personal way than just writing a big check to a funeral director."[51] Families should have the right to care for their own dead if they want to. Unfortunately, as a society, we have lost the common knowledge of how to care for the dead, so the growing availability of home funeral guides to help families is a welcome development. Home funerals, like green burials, are growing in popularity because people like having more control over and engagement with their deaths and the deaths of their loved ones.

Donating Your Body to Science and Medicine[52]

What about donating your body to science or a medical school? You do something generous and honorable when you leave your body to science and medicine. It's a meaningful way to leave a lasting legacy. Moreover, it can be a cost-effective alternative to conventional burial or flame cremation, as many medical institutions cover the costs associated with the donation process.

The best and easiest way to donate your body to science is to arrange it beforehand. Most people sign up with their state anatomy board before death. This process is easy for your loved ones because the anatomy board picks up the body and takes care of the death certificate, so a funeral director does not need to be involved.

* * * * *

This chapter explored the body-disposition options you face when thinking about your own death and the choices you face when dealing with the body disposition of a loved one. The next logical topic to consider is how to commemorate and celebrate the life of a person who has died. You need to think about this for yourself when your time comes, and you will have to think about it for a loved one who dies.

CHAPTER 11

Memorial Services, Eulogies, and Obituaries

It's appropriate for all of us to plan our own funeral or memorial service. Doing so is a generous gift to surviving loved ones, who will appreciate the help and feel happy they're giving us what we want.

The primary purpose of a funeral or memorial service is to celebrate the deceased and comfort the living. In designing the event, the desires of both the family and the deceased person need to be considered. This chapter discusses ways to commemorate and celebrate a person's life. It also advises on obituaries and eulogies.

You Don't Have to Follow the Conventional Rules

The goal is to find a meaningful way to honor someone you love and admire and say goodbye to him in a way that respects his uniqueness. You don't have to use a cleric or funeral director and follow standard burial conventions. You don't have to acquiesce to a traditional church service. You can create your own memorial service. The loved ones of the deceased can plan what to say, who to say it, what stories to tell, when to open the floor to others, what music to play, and whom to invite. You can see how I have done this for myself in appendix IV.

You can take control of the situation and create something worthy of the loved one who has died. You don't need to surrender to convention, as I did for my parents. We gave up control, handed everything over to third parties, spent no time with the bodies, had a church service with a pastor we didn't know, and said goodbye superficially and in a way that provided little comfort. Having a family come together to plan a memorial service might even help with grieving, as everyone focuses on the shared goal of creating something significant, memorable, and meaningful.

You may want to consider having a celebration-of-life party (even before the loved one has died); having in-home bathing of the body; keeping the body at home for a day (using ice packs to slow decomposition); not embalming; and encouraging in-home visits from other grieving friends and neighbors.

A Living Wake

Sadly, giving a eulogy is the first time some grieving people take the opportunity to express how meaningful and important another person's life has been to them. Ideally, we should express the loving sentiments of our eulogy to people *before* they die. Although unconventional, having a memorial service *before* a loved one dies (while still cognitively functioning) makes sense so they can hear the eulogies, enjoy them, and thank people. This is called a "living wake," "before death funeral," "living memorial," or "living funeral."

A family member can be the officiant, celebrant, or master of ceremonies, and the celebration can be uncomplicated and straightforward. The guests form a circle around the loved one being celebrated and who is nearing the end of life. The officiant states the ceremony's purpose and why everyone has gathered, and sets the intention. After this come some readings, music, and, if desired, prayers. The heart of the event is when participants stand up and tell loving, poignant, or funny stories about their loved one that reveal the loved one's character and life. Everyone present has a chance to say thank you and to hug the person being celebrated.

Funeral Service versus Memorial Service

A funeral service differs from a memorial service because the former usually happens with the body present. In contrast, a memorial service usually happens weeks or months after the body is cremated or buried.

A funeral service happens soon after the death, so the family may still be experiencing intense grief and shock. When the memorial service takes place, the grief may be easing, and the service can focus on celebrating the deceased's life as much as mourning the loss.

MEMORIAL SERVICE

The memorial service is a chance to remember and tell stories about a loved one who has died. Those memories from friends and family will likely be entertaining, funny, and comforting. Saying goodbye to a person with expressions of love and tenderness creates an imperishable and hallowed event that can profoundly impact the people present.

A thoughtful gift to your surviving loved ones is to suggest ideas on how they might celebrate your life at your memorial service. It's not macabre or morbid to do this, but kind and generous. You won't be there, so you want them to do whatever is best for them, but they want to do what would have pleased you, so it's helpful to give them some ideas before you die.[1]

A memorial service can be celebrated virtually anywhere, including a place of worship, a home, a hotel, a funeral home, or a park. You will want to choose a location that's both meaningful and convenient. Consider such practical issues as cost, availability, number of attendees, and accessibility. Decide if the gathering will be small or open to the community. Holding a memorial service in your home permits virtually unlimited time for visiting and sharing stories about the loved one who died. Potentially, you could welcome family and friends to a day-long celebration of the deceased, but your house may not be practical for this because of its size, parking availability, and other factors.

You might want to consider asking a family member to run the service. Others close to the deceased might do the readings or share personal testimonials and stories. Children or grandchildren can hand out programs. A printed program can feature a photo of the deceased on the cover and a brief biography or tribute on the back. The service, including the music and the readings, can be outlined inside the program. Guests find such a program helpful.

PUTTING THE FUN IN FUNERALS

Funerals shouldn't necessarily be somber, no-laughter affairs. Plenty of funeral and memorial services today feature funny remembrances, instructions for guests to dress in the Hawaiian shirts the deceased loved, and so on.

Invariably, one of the most poignant parts of a memorial service is when people share moving, funny, or insightful stories about the person who has died. These tributes are often called eulogies.

EULOGIES

Eulogies sum up a life, share warm memories, honor the deceased, and celebrate what the person has meant to everyone in attendance. Being invited to give a eulogy is a great honor and not one to be taken lightly. Most people have a powerful desire to honor and celebrate those who have died. It's consoling to bid farewell to loved ones with a meaningful and gracious eulogy that expresses love and gratitude for a full and purposeful life that is now complete.[2]

In her book *Remembrances and Celebrations*, author Jill Werman Harris writes that delivering a eulogy is self-defining because we learn something about the eulogist.[3] Too many eulogies fulfill what is proper or socially prescribed without doing true justice to the uniqueness and the distinctive essence of the person who has died. The eulogist might briefly summarize the person's life—pivotal events, important relationships, achievements, and interests—and then add a few favorite memories. Stories and anecdotes are eulogy gold, especially when they include humor and levity.

Consider including eccentricities, quirks, beloved sayings, favorite jokes, nuggets of wisdom, endearing habits, and whimsical views. What distinguished the dead person? What were her deeply held values and principles? What did she care about? What was her philosophy of life?

CANDOR MATTERS

A eulogy should accurately describe the life of the deceased and what that life was like. It should be honest and not misrepresent the person. We all have faults, and we all have stumbled and made mistakes. Most of these do not belong in a eulogy, but to imply perfection is misleading. Similarly, underplaying the person's virtues and failing to fully account for the blessings she brought to her family and society would make no sense.

People want to know who the deceased truly was and why he was loved. I was impressed when my niece Georgie, in the eulogy she gave for her dad, spoke openly about her father's (i.e., my brother's) alcoholism and then described his brave efforts to fight it. Candor is good if it doesn't go overboard and upset other survivors or family members. Openness, within reason and good judgment, can bring a eulogy alive, evince sympathy for the deceased, and enhance the person's standing and reputation. You want to convey the nuanced richness and breadth of the person.

A eulogy is often the most meaningful part of a memorial service. The eulogy should last no more than fifteen minutes for maximum impact; usually, five minutes is plenty. Write your eulogy down so you don't ramble. Stay away from potentially embarrassing material. Focus on the person who died, not on yourself. A meaningful and thoughtful eulogy is a labor of love. Appendix III provides an example of a eulogy. It's the one I gave for my beloved twin brother, Jonathan, in October 2022, after his sudden and unexpected death.

Draft Notes for Your Own Eulogy

Jot down notes on what might be included in your own eulogy. You should do this long before you are close to dying. Your family will appreciate the help. They want to do an outstanding job. They are drafting something about you that will summarize your life, something future generations will depend on for information about you. Just as death cleaning is a gift to your surviving family, leaving notes about your eulogy is a gift. It makes it more likely you'll get the eulogy you deserve.

Otherwise, eulogists may say anything they please, which may likely be about your career and the organizations you worked for. But will they describe what you were *really* like? What your character and personality were like? If you want people to know what you thought and who you were, jot down some notes. Your eulogist will thank you.

OBITUARIES

Providing notes for your obituary is a good idea, too, and your surviving loved ones will be grateful for the help. An obituary is an announcement that a loved one has died. It alerts others about the details of any viewing, memorial, funeral, and burial services, shares information about the person's life, and serves as a record for future generations. As you plan your loved one's obituary, check with the funeral home (if you're using a funeral home). It may have a guide for obituary writing. It also may have an online platform on which to place a digital obituary and invite people to share memories.

There is no "correct" way to draft an obituary. The first step is to collect the necessary raw information. Start with an announcement of the death that identifies the person and states that the loved one has died. Include the person's age, hometown, date of death, and the names of the person's parents and surviving family members. You might add that the death was sudden or came after a long illness and include the time and place of death. If true, you could add that the person was surrounded by family.

You will want to include a summary of the person's life. This is a way to honor the person and the meaning his life held, but it also helps other people remember him.[4] Reach out to people who knew the person so they can contribute information and ideas. It's usual to include the person's job and career information, if it applies, and any educational achievements. It is also customary to add a brief word about the person's community activities and hobbies.

If the obituary is intended to be published as a "news" (not paid) obituary in a newspaper, the more prominent newspapers require a cause of death. A "sudden" death or "long illness" does not suffice. So few "news" obituaries run in newspapers today that families are left to buy expensive paid ones. In those, you can say almost anything you want and don't have to list a cause of death.[5]

* * * * *

This chapter discussed the best ways to celebrate and commemorate the life of a loved one who has died. Closely associated with death and memorial services is the painful issue of grief and mourning. We turn to this topic next.

CHAPTER 12

Grief and Mourning

COMING TO TERMS WITH DEATH CAN BE INTENSE, TOUGH, AND CHALlenging. Grief is the internal experience of loss, while mourning is its expression. Together, they are called bereavement. This chapter discusses grief and mourning, what they are, how to deal with them, why they often are unbearably painful, and how to get help when needed. We'll discuss grief that loved ones feel and grief we feel about our own lives.

Grief is what we think and feel on the inside when someone we love dies, such as loneliness, panic, pain, yearning, and anxiety. Everyone grieves in her own way. No set path is "correct." Realizing that may help mollify the anguish. Grief can happen in many forms. Sometimes, waves of tormenting despair permeate every part of the body, and churning, complex emotions may make the grieving person almost catatonic. A grieving person may feel deep sadness, anger, isolation, abandonment, depression, exhaustion, and fatigue.

Mourning, the outward expression of grief, includes tangible and observable actions, such as crying, talking about the loss, journaling, writing letters, attending a funeral or memorial service, wearing black or other symbolic clothing, and engaging in rituals or customs associated with the culture or religion of the individual. Mourning often presents an added challenge because people tend to be uneasy with outward expressions of grief. But mourning serves several purposes, including providing a socially accepted outlet for grief, expressing feelings, and facilitating support from others. It helps individuals acknowledge the reality of the loss and begin the healing process.

LOVE AND GRIEF

The 1993 film *The Shadowlands*, starring Anthony Hopkins and Debra Winger, is about author and philosopher C. S. Lewis's love for the American poet Joy Gresham in the early 1950s. The film explores the question, "Why love if loving hurts so much?" Gresham and Lewis discuss whether love is worth the suffering, pain, and grief that hits when death looms, and Gresham says, "The pain now is part of the happiness then."

Grief and love are inextricably tied together. To live well means to love. To love means to feel gratitude and deep appreciation for another and thus to suffer one day from the piercing agony of grief. Grief is love's fury at the damage inflicted by death. All who love intensely must, at some point, bear the pain of loss. Suffering is the natural response to loss. Author Barbara Coombs Lee writes, "Such suffering can be one of the most profound experiences in a fully-lived life."[1] Author and death-care expert Barbara Karnes, RN, says, "It is important to accept grief and the hurt and pain within us and not try to push it away, hide it, or deny it."[2]

THE POWER OF GRIEF

We long to be healthy, spend time with loved ones, and finish projects we care about. We love those close to us and never want to be separated from them. We don't want to be extinguished by death. We fear losing everything we have. Losing someone we are closely attached to is life-transforming because it can shake our identity to its roots. Who is a husband without his wife? A daughter without her parents? A parent without her child? While death is a natural part of life, it's nonetheless shattering.

When author Joan Didion wrote *The Year of Magical Thinking*, she attempted to make sense of what happened to her when her husband, John Gregory Dunne, suddenly died and their only daughter, Quintana, died nineteen months later. She describes grief as coming "in waves, paroxysms, sudden apprehensions that weaken the knees and blind the eyes and obliterate the dailiness of life."[3] A single person has died, but the whole world seems empty and meaningless. The grieving person feels shock, a sense of disbelief, and numbness. Didion wrote, "Grief turns out to be a place none of us know until we reach it."[4]

ACUTE GRIEF RESPONSES

Acute grief is painful, overwhelming, and intense. Some of the commonly felt grief responses, as reported by many bereaved people, include the following:[5]

1. A range of emotions, including sadness and depression, anxiety, guilt or anger about things said or done (or things not said or done), gratitude that your loved one's suffering is over, denial that the death actually happened, and numbness and shock;

2. A range of sensations, including extreme forgetfulness, trouble concentrating, insomnia, excessive tiredness, heaviness in the chest, tightness in the throat, loss of appetite, mood swings, and sensing your loved one's presence; and

3. A range of behaviors, including crying at unexpected times, overeating, undereating, wandering aimlessly, exploding in anger, telling and retelling stories about the dead person, questioning spiritual and religious beliefs, and overactivity (keeping busy to try to avoid this new reality).

These are all natural and normal grief responses. As the nurses and other staff at Montgomery Hospice and Prince George's Hospice say, you are not going crazy when you feel them. You are grieving because you dared to love.[6]

The goal is not to stop feeling the painful loss of a loved one but to come to terms with it, find new purpose and meaning in life, and eventually reconnect with healthy daily activities. A new relationship with the deceased loved one evolves into something that allows you to reengage with life.

GRIEVING PEOPLE WANT TO BE UNDERSTOOD

Grief is so powerful that, in addition to its emotional and mental dimensions, it has a physical dimension. Our bodies scream with pain; our stomachs knot tightly. When a loved one dies, we realize, to our horror, that we will no longer see that person alive. We know we are vulnerable to death, too, and the delusion that we are safe from death fades, intensifying our grief.

When we grieve, we try to understand a world that has had its meaning broken and crushed by loss and death. It helps to have someone with us who fully understands the enormity of our loss without downplaying it or pointing out silver linings. Grieving people often yearn for someone to listen to their suffering and their story without receiving shallow advice and bromides.[7]

GRIEF IS NOT A DISEASE

As we age, we'll all suffer losses beyond those of friends and loved ones, including losses of prestige, status, income, strength, flexibility, height, eyesight, hearing, bladder and bowel control, the long-term family house, and the identities tied to our careers. A sense of loss leads to feelings of grief, and it's a healthy, natural emotion. If we love life as we should, then loss is part of that lived experience, and we are going to grieve when loss occurs. We should not think of grief as a problem to be solved.

When we think of grief as a disease that needs to be cured, we're pathologizing grief and thinking of it as wrong in some way. In reality, it's an emotion (or, more accurately, a hurricane of emotions) that we should embrace as the price for living a rich life. For most people, a sense of acceptance and normalcy begins to edge back within a year or so after the death of a loved one. If this doesn't happen, some therapists might identify your suffering as complicated grief.

COMPLICATED GRIEF

In early 2022, psychiatry formally introduced a new pathological designation called complicated or "prolonged grief." The fifth edition of the *Diagnostic and Statistical Manual of Mental Disorders* (D.S.M.-5) states that "prolonged grief" is a mental disorder. The manual defines this illness as an intense pain lasting a year after a loss and an inability to resume past activities. Including prolonged and complicated grief in D.S.M.-5 allows a diagnosis and enables insurance payments to cover treatment for times when grieving people are unable to function and reengage with life.

Some observers find this designation problematic and even alarming because they argue that grief that lasts more than a year may be completely normal, rational behavior and should not be treated as a disease and something that needs to be "cured."[8] After all, if your teenage daughter dies from suicide, who has the right to say to you, "You should get over your grief within a year." That would be ludicrous. The grief may last a lifetime, and that is understandable.

But if, after a year or more, a grieving person is severely depressed, guilt-stricken, or has other intense and perhaps harmful symptoms, getting help from a professional therapist specializing in grief may be wise. For the most part, grief is a natural consequence of losing someone we love and realizing that all the possibilities we had for that person have vanished.

REMORSE, REGRETS, AND UNFINISHED BUSINESS

Grief is often made worse because we regret shameful behavior or feel remorse over never having the courage or common sense to say "I'm sorry" or "I love you" to loved ones before they die. Unfinished business and "open loops" (unfulfilled commitments or incomplete tasks) can exacerbate feelings of intense sadness and loss. The abolitionist and novelist Harriet Beecher Stowe writes, "The bitterest tears shed over graves are for words left unsaid and deeds left undone."[9] Similarly, author Sarah Murray writes, "Grief, it seems to me, is often bound up in unfinished business—remorse for bad behavior or regret for the things we never got to say to those we've lost."[10]

When a loved one dies, there can be "open loops." No relationship is perfect. Author and nurse Barbara Karnes recommends that one way to deal with open loops or unfinished business is to put our thoughts on paper and write a letter to the deceased saying all the things that weren't said (but perhaps should have been) when they were alive. Writing helps sort out our feelings and brings order and clarity to our roiling thoughts. Some people find grieving a positive experience because it's time to fill one's mind with happy memories of the deceased and a profound appreciation for the deceased's life.

Holding on to grief may be a way to keep a lost loved one close and ever-present, but, for most people, time does bring relief from the piercing pain of grief. In a sense, the dead are still alive because they live on within us and show up in words and humor that bring the deceased to mind. Loving memories give us life after death. As I wrote in chapter 5, after we die, we can live again in others by what we gave. We all die, but our character lives on in our loved ones and friends, and knowing this can help ease the pain of grief.

ELISABETH KÜBLER-ROSS AND THE STAGES OF GRIEF

The Swiss-American psychiatrist Elisabeth Kübler-Ross is often credited with discovering the five stages of grief, but this is inaccurate. She worked with people who were dying, not grieving. Her five stages—denial, anger, bargaining, depression, and acceptance—are coping mechanisms for people facing a terrible situation. Kübler-Ross did not claim these stages came in some neat order. She said they overlapped, went in a different order for different people, repeatedly reappeared at other times, and were sometimes experienced simultaneously.

That such coping mechanisms are needed is not surprising. Unease about death defines us as humans. As far as we know, no animals besides humans contemplate their finitude and fleeting nature, though other species, such as elephants, display behaviors consistent with grief about death.

Why wouldn't we be anxious and upset about death and develop coping mechanisms like bargaining and acceptance? Death means physical extinction, no small matter. Grief lasts as long as needed, which occasionally means a lifetime. We have lost what we most desperately want to hang on to and hold tight, and that loss is devastating.

DAVID KESSLER AND THE SIXTH STAGE OF GRIEF

David Kessler, a grief expert who worked closely with Elisabeth Kübler-Ross, makes the case in his book *Finding Meaning* that searching for meaning is a crucial sixth stage of the healing process. In this sixth stage, we acknowledge that grief will never really end (even though it may lessen in intensity over time), but that, if we move fully into this stage and search for meaning, it will "allow us to transform grief into something else, something rich and fulfilling."[11]

David Kessler says this can take many forms, such as finding gratitude for the time spent with deceased loved ones, finding ways to honor and commemorate them, or realizing the transitory nature of life and how precious it is and making that a catalyst for a life transformation. He says meaning comes through finding a way to sustain your love for the dead person while you move forward with your life.

Grieving is important, and a healthy person allows the pain of grief to settle in and take its time to get resolved. As mentioned earlier, grieving deeply when you lose someone you cherish is part of living a rewarding life.

ANTICIPATORY GRIEF

A few of us will die suddenly because of an accident, sudden illness, assault, or another reason. But most of us will die slowly. In that situation, grief often starts well before death occurs. When patients first receive a worrying, or perhaps shattering, diagnosis, revealing that they are facing a serious illness, the immediate losses—of hope, energy, independence, freedom, and a pain-free body—can cause the onset of anticipatory grief. We fear being dependent on others and losing our self-reliance. Of course, the same anticipatory grief hits those who love and care for the afflicted patient. Dr. BJ Miller and Shoshana Berger point out that anticipatory grief can be helpful "as a kind of practice for what is to come."[12]

DISENFRANCHISED GRIEF

People sometimes feel disenfranchised grief, that is, grief that is unacknowledged because others do not assess it as valid. This is unfair and heartless. For example, hospice volunteers who grow close to their dying patients deserve sympathy and compassion for the legitimate grief they feel when their patient dies. People who lose a pet or an ex-spouse or who feel bonded to a deceased celebrity can feel intense grief, which is as valid as any other type of grief.

GRIEF EXPERIENCED DIFFERENTLY BY MEN AND WOMEN

People sometimes claim that men and women grieve differently. Grief experts say, however, that grief has less to do with gender and more to do with our preferred, innate grieving style. Dealing with the death of a loved one is extraordinarily difficult, whether you are a man or woman or if you self-identify with another gender variation. You have to accept the reality of the loss, process the pain of grief, adjust to a world without the loved one in it, and then find an enduring connection with the deceased while reengaging with life.

SECONDARY LOSSES

In addition to the loss of a loved one who has died, a grieving person has worrying and sometimes unbearable secondary losses, including the loss of dreams for the future, a support system, identity, confidence, financial security, and income.

Grieving is always hard and challenging, but certain things make it harder. As mentioned, guilt, remorse, and regrets make the road rockier. Other examples include being highly dependent on the deceased, experiencing other deaths or losses, or having a mental illness.

The systemic stigma of discussing grief, death, and dying is a troubling factor as well. Western culture does a terrible job of normalizing conversations on these topics. Recognizing that we live in a system that is reluctant to broach the issues makes it harder for those grieving.

SUDDEN, UNANTICIPATED, AND UNATTENDED DEATH

Grieving may be harsher if the death was traumatic, violent, or unexpected, if the death was by suicide, or if you bear some responsibility for the death, such as in a gun accident or a car crash.[13]

Examples of unexpected death (compared to death from a drawn-out terminal illness) include deaths from plane accidents, car crashes, violence, suicide, terrorism, and acute diseases. Handling the grief ignited by a sudden and unexpected death is extremely challenging.

One of the most harrowing deaths to deal with is death from suicide. Medical journalist Jane Brody writes that grieving survivors "typically receive far less support from others than if the death had occurred as a result of cancer or a traffic accident, for example."[14]

Too often, says Brody, death from suicide is viewed as a death people bring on themselves and thus a death that is perhaps less worthy of being mourned. But that hardly makes it less agonizing or traumatic for the survivors. Mourners of deaths from suicide are no less deserving of compassion and empathy.

BEREAVEMENT SUPPORT GROUPS

Hospice agencies offer bereavement services to those grieving, whether or not the deceased family member was signed up with them. Hospice organizations can also help people find appropriate bereavement support groups that provide protected places to share thoughts, reflections, and anxieties without feeling self-conscious or judged.

Bereavement support groups are for anyone experiencing pain and suffering because of a death. They are for people in anguish over their loss and for anyone who has lost someone and wants to talk about it. Bereavement support groups offer a place to share feelings and emotions that may be tearing the grieving person apart. They are places where those who share the searing experience of a severe loss can gather and find strength in simply meeting and talking.

HOW TO TALK TO THE GRIEVING

The advice in chapter 9 on how to talk to those ill and dying is germane to talking with the grieving. When comforting someone who is grieving, it's essential to listen, to steer clear of platitudes (like "she is in a better place" or "everything happens for a reason"), and to share stories and memories of the deceased person.

My friend Ann Bennet lost her beloved husband, Philip, six years ago. She misses him terribly and thinks about him every day. What has made her grief worse is that barely anyone mentions his name anymore. Ann says sadly, "It sometimes feels as if Philip never existed in their lives."[15] Those grieving want to know that their loved one won't be forgotten and that their lives had meaning.

GRIEF AND BUSYNESS

It takes significant time to deal with all the paperwork when someone dies and to wind down the life of the deceased. The drudgery ranges from canceling a driver's license to notifying the board of elections. Amid all this necessary busyness, grieving—fully grieving—can get neglected. While understandable, this is not healthy.

GRIEF RITUALS

The subject of grief rituals is vast and beyond the scope of this book. There has been much scholarship and research on the role of grief rituals and their importance.[16] During the Civil War, wearing black clothing when someone died was a long-accepted custom to show respect for the deceased. Grief rituals like wearing black help to ease the pain of grief and loss. Judaism has many grief rituals, but, as a general rule, Americans have few death rituals that are widely shared. As a society, we are the poorer for that paucity.

LEARNING FROM JUDAISM

There is a lot to learn from Judaism. A wise insight about grief comes from Rabbi Earl Grollman, who said, "Grief is not a disorder, a disease, or a sign of weakness. It is an emotional, physical, and spiritual necessity, the price you pay for love. The only cure for grief is to grieve." The fundamental message of Judaism about death and grief is that we are not alone and should not feel alone. Every custom of Jewish mourning and comforting has, at its core, the motivation to surround those who are dying and those who will grieve with a supportive, caring community.

While coping with grief can heighten one's feeling of aloneness, the Jewish approach places grief in the community and among family and friends. Comforters are obligated to tend to the needs of mourners. For instance, since a Jewish family sitting shiva (seven days of mourning following a death) should not be burdened by having to prepare meals, it's the community's responsibility to feed them.

Shiva is a Hebrew word meaning "seven" and refers to a seven-day period of formalized mourning by the deceased's immediate family. Shiva was traditionally done for seven days, although many Reform and other Jews now sit shiva for three days, and some for one day.

REENGAGING WITH LIFE

When the agony of grief eventually eases a little, as it does for most people, one might consider how best to cherish the memories of the loved one who has died and ponder how those grieving can slowly reengage with life. Grieving and mourning are distinct from recalling and celebrating the life of a loved one. How do you keep them, in a sense, alive and continue to draw strength from them? How do you develop rituals that allow for remembrance and healing?

Ideas include acknowledging their birthdays and "deathdays," telling stories about them, cooking their favorite recipes, sharing old photos of them with friends and family, and recognizing when their example inspires you to behave generously and admirably.

Author and friend Diane MacEachern says,

> I have told my kids that when I die, they can see me in beautiful gardens, the ocean, and Nature. I've encouraged them to fill their house with flowers on Mother's Day or my birthday. I will sometimes say to them, "Long after I'm gone, I want you to remember . . ." and give them maxims and sayings I hope they keep close.

> I'm pulling together a couple of picture books for them, in addition to the legacy letter I'm writing for each of them. One is a book of pictures of them with me, at all ages, starting in utero. Another is a book that highlights our many travels together. They'll be fun to give them when I'm alive, and I think they'll enjoy having them when I'm dead.

Diane also models this for them. She will call her children on their grandparents' birthdays, remind them they were wonderful people, and tell them funny or endearing stories about them.

* * * * *

As we approach the end of this book about achieving a good death, I want to devote the epilogue to exploring ways to reimagine death and think about it more constructively rather than letting it fill us with anxiety. We must make it a topic we can discuss easily, positively, and usefully.

Epilogue

Reimagining Death and Dying

I HOPE THIS BOOK HAS HELPED TO GIVE YOU THE KNOWLEDGE AND skills needed to achieve a good and peaceful death. As we have seen, dying well takes preparation and planning, and living well is one of the best ways to increase your chances of attaining a good death. There is an art to dying well. It's something people can get skilled at achieving. As I wrote in the Preface, death is inevitable, but dying badly is not.

In his book *American: Beyond Our Grandest Notions*, author and former TV host Chris Matthews argues that America is a nation built on independence, individualism, and self-reliance.[1] It makes sense, then, that we would insist on making our own decisions regarding death and dying. Americans don't like others, especially those who appear imperious or arrogant, telling them what to do. Decisions about our bodies and end-of-life choices must be made by the person dying (or the person's health-care agent) and not by doctors or clerics.

A long life as a healthy person is a pleasure, but, for too many of us, this enjoyable interval is followed by a gradual, lingering, and painful death. This book has shown that there is a different, gentler, and more humane approach that can lead to a more comfortable dying process and eventual death. The goal is to make death and dying less daunting and more responsive to the dying person's wishes. Sometimes, there are more important goals than delaying death as long as possible, regardless of the quality of life.

The bioethicist Dr. Ezekiel Emanuel is one doctor who has given much thought to the connection between living well and dying well.

In an essay published in *The Atlantic* in October 2014, entitled "Why I Hope to Die at 75," Emanuel argues that patients should no longer seek curative help from doctors after age seventy-five because they should avoid burdening family members and society. I disagree with his arbitrary choice of seventy-five (why not eighty-five or even older if you are in robust health), but, undoubtedly, there will come a time for each of us when our frailty, quality of life, chronic illness, or incapacity to function will lead us to allow only palliative care and to refuse to accept last-ditch medical treatments.

Emanuel sets a good example of the type of intentional approach to death and dying that is sensible and wise. He has thought about it, is not approaching it haphazardly, and is looking ahead and trying to make sense of a perplexing challenge. He's living by his values, doing what is best for him, and discussing his wishes with his family. This is what we must all do.

We get old and die. The people we love will die. Regardless of our life experiences, income, religion, cultural customs, or skin color, our lives all have finitude, brevity, and the certainty of loss. We are part of nature, and death is natural. Grasping this truth helps us value each precious moment, knowing it's a temporary blessing. Not talking about death only leads to suffering and anguish. We must face our fear of death head-on and be willing to say aloud and with conviction, "I am mortal and one day will die." This is the start of learning the art of dying well and having a good death. The dead and dying teach us something we resist learning—that we will die someday.

We should live full, purposeful lives *because of* death, not despite death. Despite how fleeting life is, we must embrace the truth of our impermanence and cherish our life's profound beauty and preciousness. Our brief life can enrich us if we choose to let it. Poet Emily Dickinson writes, "That it will never come again is what makes life so sweet."[2] It's wise to embrace the transitory nature of our lives and use that knowledge to help us improve our lives and our deaths. Our very transience—our realization of how little time we each have on Earth—can lead us to think about why we're here and what we can do to make the most of our lives.

So many of us leave few traces of our existence. We skim through life and live shallow, mediocre, and haphazard lives. Sometimes, when a person dies, there isn't much to point to as worth remembering. The fear of not being worth remembering aggravates our fear of death. One way to reduce the terror and dread of death is to live fully so we can feel good about our lives and have few regrets when we die. We can apologize to our estranged sibling, thank a parent for all he has done for us, and say a loving goodbye to a grandparent.

This realization of potential future regrets can also be what psychiatrist Irvin Yalom calls an "awakening experience" that teaches us to live fully. An awakening event can incentivize us to reinvent our lives and not be so fearful of dying and death.[3] As discussed in chapter 2, we can learn to live well and stop accumulating regrets. An awakening experience can catalyze a deep awareness of our temporary nature and help us to realize that we should not squander our time.

Only when we appreciate how little time we have with our loved ones do we begin to see that we must make the most of that time. As Yalom writes, "The way to value life, the way to feel compassion for others, the way to love anything with greatest depth is to be aware that these experiences are destined to be lost."[4] As we approach the end of our lives and ruminate more often on our death and what dying means, the need to marshal the best parts of our character to deal with the challenge becomes more important. My friend and naturalist Meredith Taylor says, "Life is too sweet and precious to waste a single day or hour. Accordingly, my husband and I stay busy doing things we love."[5]

Based on what we think matters (which will vary from person to person), we need to develop a vision of how we want to complete our lives. In chapter 2, I analyzed why creating a vision for our lives is vital.[6] We must also develop a vision for our dying and death. You can see mine in appendix I and appendix IV. We strive for meaning, dignity, and purpose in our lives, and we can bring that same intentionality to our deaths. Embracing our mortality, completing an advance directive with a dementia provision, and talking with our loved ones about what we want at the end of our lives can help us achieve a good death while invigorating how we live now.

We should be grateful for death rather than fearing it because it provokes us to consider profound questions about our lives, questions that might otherwise remain dormant. Author, aphorist, and quotation expert Dr. Mardy Grothe says, "For some, the idea of death represents a final curtain; for others, it's more like an alarm clock, awakening us to all that remains to be done."[7] We need to ask spiritual questions about the end of life. By spiritual, I'm referring to those things that give life meaning and purpose.[8] Contemplating death leads us to ask questions about the purpose and meaning of life. Asking such questions and eschewing glib, facile answers can add depth and richness to our lives.

Author Dr. Katharine Esty asked a large number of older people what lessons they had learned from their long lives about what really matters. She discovered that no one mentioned accomplishments, power, fame, wealth, and looking good. Instead, people said the importance of family, following your dreams, serving others, living in the present, and remembering that relationships matter more than anything else.[9]

Death is inevitable, but concluding that life has no purpose is wrong. Facing our finitude boldly and courageously while creating meaning in our lives (thereby making the most of them) is a challenge worth accepting. By bravely accepting our impermanence, we can live fuller, larger, and more colorful lives. By acknowledging death, we strengthen our lives; by denying death, we weaken and shrink them. To die is a smaller tragedy than the tragedy that happens when a person does not live the best, most fulfilling life possible. The most frightening aspect of death may be that, as it arrives, we might discover, to our horror, in Thoreau's words, that we haven't lived.

Death's centrality to virtually all philosophies and religions is no accident. By not embracing death, like most people with death-denying attitudes, we unthinkingly reject the purpose it can give us. When people live shallow, empty lives, constantly distracted by trifles, it's because death seems far off and unreal. We assume the essential things that must be done (like being kind, generous, and compassionate) can be postponed. Awareness of death and that it can occur at any time has a clarifying power. When we face our mortality, instead of hiding from it, we stop being willing to waste time on frivolous activities and toxic relationships.

If we lived every day as if death were only a few days away, our main challenge would be expressing love to people. Impending mortality gives urgency to expressions of appreciation, caring, and gratitude. Confronted by death, we naturally want to strengthen relationships with those we love and care about. We also try to make sense of our life experiences and to feel like a part of something (such as a noble cause) more significant and enduring than ourselves.

We tend to see ourselves as the center of the universe, forgetting how utterly unimportant and small we are in the context of the universe and vast geologic time. Yet, to the people who love us, we *are* important. As human beings, we have deep inner feelings, are amazingly expressive, can love and show empathy and compassion, are curious, and love to learn. We also experience feelings of awe and transcendence, have consciousness and scruples, have epiphanies and revelations, and have yearnings to live an exemplary and honorable life.

Paradoxically, despite being what might be termed godlike, we die like any other animal, and the world goes on without us. No one knows the answer to this paradox. Still, we can confidently say that the best way to face death is to grab life by the lapels and engage in it—engaging in those very activities that make us so godlike and so unlike other animals.

To confront our death is to be fully alive because it makes us cherish mundane and quotidian delights, like a simple act of kindness or generosity, that we might otherwise take for granted. Knowing that we have lived a good life can comfort us when dying. The author and psychiatrist Irvin Yalom writes, "The greater the sense of unlived life, the greater the terror of death."[10]

Tolstoy's novella *The Death of Ivan Ilych*, published in 1886, describes how forty-five-year-old Ivan Ilych realizes he is dying badly (from some unnamed, untreatable disease) because he has lived badly.[11] Ilych's whole life, as author and surgeon Atul Gawande puts it, "revolves mostly around petty concerns of social status."[12] Tolstoy points out that Ilych's intense suffering is exacerbated because no one will talk with him about his dying. Everyone around him pretends he's sick and will get better, but Ilych knows he's doomed and desperately wants to talk about the mess he's in. The fact that he has such poor relationships with most of his caregivers reflects the poor quality of his life.

Doctors, family members, and patients sometimes seem to conspire silently to deny the reality that a patient is dying and refuse to acknowledge it openly. But palliative care doctor B. J. Miller writes, "It has always seemed to me that dying people know they are dying and are relieved when those around them can share that truth."[13] Many people's fears about death are fueled partly by their despair and disappointment at never fully living and living far below their potential. With time running out, the fear of failing at life becomes unbearable. We are haunted by the feeling that we have let down ourselves and our loved ones and that it didn't have to be that way. The key message of *The Death of Ivan Ilych* is that awareness of an unlived, unused life can be terrifying and disturbing. In his book *Death Over Dinner*, author and death expert Michael Hebb reports, "Some hospice nurses have shared that patients with unfinished emotional business suffer the greatest physical pain during the dying process."[14]

We've talked about how an unfulfilled life can exacerbate our terror of death. A good death is not being terrified. For example, some people resolve as they approach death to model how to face it with grit and grace for their families and friends. Having a purpose (or, if you like, a mission) up until the very end helps to provide life with meaning, which in turn helps to create a sense of serenity and well-being. Death reminds us that we have only one chance at life, one brief moment in the sun. Thus, we should live as fully and exuberantly as possible, favoring the important over the trivial. People living meaningful, significant, and purposeful lives tend to have less fear of death and dying.

Facing death with grace, dignity, and courage becomes a little easier if we have lived well and believe that our influence and impact extend beyond our deaths, perhaps through our children, our values, our art, or our volunteer activities. Authors and professors Jeff Greenberg, Sheldon Solomon, and Tom Pyszczynski, in their book *On the Role of Death in Life: The Worm at the Core*, write that we must "really grasp that being mortal, while terrifying, can also make our lives sublime by infusing us with courage, compassion, and concern for future generations."[15] Such an understanding can lead us to seek enduring significance through our good works.

We strive for immortality—for ways to overcome death—through our children and grandchildren, the legacy letters and ethical wills we compose, our religious beliefs, and our efforts to model exemplary behavior. One of the best ways to ease death anxiety is through what the author and psychiatrist Irvin Yalom calls "rippling."[16] Yalom writes, "The idea that we can leave something of ourselves . . . offers a potent answer to those who claim that meaningless inevitably flows from one's finiteness and transiency."[17] "Rippling" does not necessarily mean leaving your name on a building or a scholarship, for example, but leaving behind some nugget of wisdom, some life experience, perhaps a virtuous character, or something you taught that gives your survivors comfort, joy, and peace. As composer and lyricist Irving Berlin writes, "The song ends, but the melody lingers on."

Rippling is when your caring, gentleness, love of life, and love of laughter rub off on your friends and family and ripple into the future. It can affect and enrich people for generations and be a great comfort for those with death anxiety. When we die, we hope to leave a legacy and have our values continue in those who survive us. As Yalom says, rippling eases the potential torment of life's transience by "reminding us that something of each of us persists even though it may be unknown or imperceptible to us." As discussed in chapter 5, we die twice—first, when we take our last breath, and, second, when we are forgotten and all evidence of the rippling from our lives ceases. The brutal truth is that virtually all of us will be forgotten after five to ten generations.

There will come a time when the last living person who remembers us dies. Then, we will move from the "remembered dead" to the "truly dead." Dwelling on such a melancholic thought is futile. The better response is to redouble our efforts to live a full life. We cannot assuage the sting of death by hoping our names, reputations, and legacies will last forever because they won't. What is the most thoughtful way to react to this realization? We have no choice but to invest all we can in our singular and unique life, which means living virtuously by being kind, considerate, and generous. It means helping others and taking worthy actions that will lead to an end of life with few regrets.

The certainty of death for everyone is 100 percent. Everything we love in life will eventually be taken from us. Finding enduring love in life is hard, but what may be even harder is living with the fact that we will lose that hard-won love. Suffering is inescapable if we live and love fully, but it can be assuaged by exercising gratitude.

When former President Jimmy Carter was told he had cancer in his brain and might die very soon, friends and observers marveled at his serenity, grace, and equanimity.[18] Carter could be at ease and feel a deep calm partly because he was in the habit of feeling grateful and realizing that things could be much worse. As *The Washington Post*'s Sarah Kaufman notes, Carter's habit of being grateful when circumstances are dire is an "underestimated superpower" because it gives a person incredible resilience and mental strength.

In a sense, we all hope for something more than a good death. Ideally, we would like a beautiful death, full of meaning and reconciliations, sprinkled with sacred moments, moving last words, and shared expressions of tender love. This utopian vision of a beautiful death is rarely realized. More often, the patient is drowsy and inward-looking, struggling with the intense hard work of dying. Even worse, the detritus of dying, from pills to commodes, is everywhere. A deathbed is not often a scene that lends itself to a sense of the sacred and mysterious. Caring for a dying person can often be overwhelming, discouraging any chance of a life-affirming and uplifting exit.

Sometimes, the most we can hope for is that Dr. Ira Byock's five life tasks mentioned in chapter 2 (expressing love, thanking, forgiving, being forgiven, saying goodbye) get completed well before the final moments and that the dying person be loved, be pain-free, have few regrets, and die feeling that life has been satisfactorily completed.

More and more physicians, led by farsighted doctors like Ira Byock, acknowledge they need more training in end-of-life conversations and how to deal with death constructively. Some doctors argue that we have a moral imperative to keep patients alive regardless of how low their quality of life plummets. In contrast, increasing numbers of doctors are saying it's better morally not to prolong the dying process artificially and to allow a patient to die peacefully. Many doctors delay changing a patient's goals of care (away from attempts to cure) until a patient is close to death, so the patient misses out on the many benefits of hospice. Sometimes, it's easier for doctors to offer more medical interventions, even if they have no benefits, than to tell the patients it's time for hospice.

We want a gentle, peaceful death without futile overtreatment that causes pain, isolation, and suffering. I don't want my last conscious thought to be of doctors stabbing needles into my veins, my ribs breaking from chest compressions, and a large-bore tube thrust into my throat and lungs. That's not a good death for a person near the end of life. Dying in an ICU on a mechanical ventilator with tubes in virtually every orifice and being unable to communicate with loved ones because of intubation and ventilation is a bad death. When a patient is young and robust, such curative measures may make good sense despite their violence, but not for an old, debilitated, frail patient.

Moving away from trying to cure the disease toward a focus (as in hospice) on mitigating pain, caring for the whole person, telling patients how much we love them, and saying farewell is a better way to end a life than dying under a code blue. It is better to stop fighting for an impossible cure and die peacefully and with dignity. As author and hospice chaplain Hank Dunn points out, the decisions regarding life-prolonging procedures are not black and white.[19] There are gray areas where there can be legitimate debate. As a patient approaches the end of life, questions about ventilation, dialysis, CPR, deactivating pacemakers, antibiotics, and hospitalization may arise. In some cases, medical intervention will be warranted, and in others not. The burden of such decision-making will be eased if patients have clarified their preferences through advance directives and conversations with their health-care agent.

It's bewildering that the medical profession devotes such colossal amounts of money to applying expensive, often painful, frequently futile advanced technologies to patients near death when what patients need is relatively inexpensive: doctors who do house calls, a caring end-of-life doula, gentleness, calm, fresh diapers, no bedsores, morphine as needed, and expressions of tenderness and gratitude from loved ones, including reassurance they are loved and won't be forgotten. In *The Art of Dying Well*, Katy Butler writes, "It is widely acknowledged that in most parts of the country, the conventional medical system—at least in its approach to the aging, incurably ill, and dying—is broken."[20] In a similar vein, Hank Dunn writes,

> Preparing for a comfortable and dignified death is a shift away from the direction of most medical care given today. It is a shift away from most of the medical training our physicians receive. It is also a shift away from the mission of our hospitals, which exist primarily to cure patients.[21]

We should not impose violent medical technologies, like CPR, on people who will die soon anyway and do not deserve to suffer the pain, complications, unintended consequences, and unanticipated side effects of such medical treatments. Author and cardiologist Haider Warraich reports that a third of older Americans undergo surgery in a hospital in the last year of life, and a fifth undergo surgery in the last month.[22] We should examine the alleged benefits of such surgical procedures skeptically. Too many terminally ill patients end up in the emergency room, where they unintentionally and grudgingly endure ineffective, invasive treatments that reduce the quality of life as they die.

Losing one's memory and ability to recognize family members is worse than death. We should have the freedom to choose our own "exit strategies." A rational "exit strategy" should be legal everywhere. Anyone who has lost someone to dementia knows its brutality to the patients and their loved ones. It's barbaric to require people to go through this. We must give these patients a compassionate exit from an unimaginable trial.

My friend Grant Thompson sent a wise letter to his doctor asking him to let Grant die peacefully when the time comes. Here is what Grant wrote in part:

> I dread a drawn-out, painful, or unaware life sustained by machines, drugs, and expensive attention. My mother's mother lay unmoving and unspeaking for five long years in the 1950s. My brother struggled with Parkinson's disease, which left him often violent, incontinent, and with

periods of severe dementia. In my case, in 2007, I was medically sedated for nearly two months as I fought pneumonia. I vividly recall the period after I was awakened, unable to speak because of a breathing tube, my hands bound to the bed to prevent me from taking IV drip lines out, and fed intravenously. That period was a horror at the time and remains my worst nightmare.

Modern medicine is a miracle. But medicine (and doctors) can too easily become one's enemy at the end of life. I read of patients subjected to "heroic" measures to extend a pitiable life for a few days or weeks at the cost of hundreds of thousands of dollars, and I recoil in dread. Please don't do that to me. I don't want it!

Life is a journey with a beginning and an end. We celebrate the birth of a child as a potential gift to the future, as a being full of possibilities. Yet, for some reason, we treat death—an event as natural and inevitable as birth—as an enemy. I do not see death as something to be fought at all costs. An intentional death, uninterrupted by vain attempts to prevent what will happen to us all, is a fitting end to every life.

All patients should write a letter along these lines to their doctors. You can find the one I wrote in appendix I.

As people approach the end of their lives, they often increasingly feel new responsibilities. They want to articulate and pass on wisdom, find and shape the story of their lives, and share and record memories. They want to say sorry, thank you, and goodbye. They want to leave a legacy, to know they won't be forgotten, and to gain assurances that their surviving loved ones will do well. When doctors take actions that interfere with and disrupt a patient's ability to carry out those responsibilities, then they are failing, especially if the person only gains an extra few days in the ICU, barely conscious and attached to machines and tubes.

Central to the purpose of medicine must be the achievement of a peaceful, good death. Care for the dying should not be a peripheral or fringe activity pushed off onto palliative care and hospice doctors as an afterthought when all else has failed. Medical ethicist Daniel Callahan writes, "The goal of a peaceful death should be as much a part of the purpose of medicine as that of the promotion of good health."[23]

The propensity of both doctors and patients to deny death causes great suffering. In our current medical environment, the default approach to helping sick, older patients is the routine use of highly sophisticated technology. As mentioned earlier, older patients are put on what palliative care doctor and ICU physician Jessica Zitter calls "the end-of-life conveyor belt," in which they are artificially fed, catheterized, intubated, and—as a result—die badly.[24]

The relentless shiny offers of modern medicine seduce us into accepting barbaric drops in our quality of life as we desperately try to extend life by a few days. Geriatrician Dr. Louise Aronson writes in *Elderhood*, "It's likely that medical care harms and kills old people in ways and numbers far beyond what gets reported."[25] Patients with terminal illnesses want to prolong their lives but may not want to do this if it conflicts with other equally important goals, such as avoiding pain and suffering, telling loved ones how much they mean to them, saying goodbye, strengthening relationships with family members, not being a burden on their caregivers, finishing projects, remaining alert, and getting to the point where they feel their lives are complete. Patients want to optimize their health and well-being according to their values and preferences. At the end of life, that may mean prolonging life, but not always.

The loss of function (mental, physical, emotional) that comes with the dying process shrinks our bodies, characters, and personalities. It can be a slow torture. Our loved ones struggle to recognize the person we used to be. Our decrepitude, debilitation, and disabilities weaken and undercut our ability to live with purpose and meaning. As death approaches, a patient's condition can be so bad that dying may be worse than death for them. For example, if they require 24/7 care, are bedridden, have bowel and bladder incontinence, need intubation and mechanical ventilation, have a feeding (PEG) tube, or are confused and agitated, the patient may find those conditions torturous and unbearable, especially if such conditions continue for days or weeks or months.

A patient may find it impossible to find any benefits in those circumstances and may prefer the option of being dead. People want to be the authors of their own lives, control what happens to their bodies, shape their own story (and not have it shaped for them by doctors), and live in a way that provides meaning, even at the end of life. At the same time, we should not stop living with intention and purpose because doctors tell us we have a terminal illness. If we're in hospice, we must remember that the purpose of hospice is not to help us die but to help us live fully until we die.

We must reinvent our thinking around end-of-life care. As a nation, we need to do more to help terminally ill patients end their suffering with the aid of a doctor. Patients don't want to lose control of their lives as they near death and want to have meaningful interactions with their loved ones as long as possible.

Humans might be the only animals aware of their finitude, but they lack the right to a merciful death, such as what we can offer to beloved pets. On March 1, 2022, the following searing letter from Robert Macht of Baltimore appeared in the *New York Times*:

> My father, Philip, killed himself by shooting himself in the head on November 11th 2011. He was 82. He asked me to kill him. I refused. I told him that I would go to jail if I killed him. He was not diagnosed with a terminal illness or a mental illness. Question: Should there have been an option for him to peacefully make an appointment for his own death? I think it's possible, that if he had had that option, he would have been more relaxed about whatever medical horrors may lay ahead for him, and he would not have chosen suicide at that time.

In the past, patients would die from any number of problems, but now, modern medicine can keep people from dying for decades. However, more and more of us are questioning this development. What is the purpose of doctors and nurses keeping patients alive if they are in intense pain, life is no longer worth living, their quality of life is appalling, and they want to hasten their death gently? An emotionally and mentally capable patient should have the right to request death when her life descends irreversibly to a subhuman level and has painfully lingered on for too long.

The way our society has failed to protect dying people from unwanted, unnecessary, and unendurable suffering is a crime. Everyone should have the right to the death he wants, whether a lingering death prolonged as long as possible or a hastened death to avoid hopelessness and unrelievable anguish. In the face of irreparable and irremediable health conditions that severely diminish a patient's autonomy and quality of life, patients should take charge of the process and hasten death if that's what they want to do, rather than let doctors' treatment plans determine the timing and experience of death.

The right to die peacefully is not a constitutional right, but perhaps it should be. People should have the right to choose to die when they are terminally ill. For decades, activist and author Derek Humphry has argued that "freedom to die in a manner of our own choosing is the ultimate personal and civil liberty." He writes, "To every person their own way of death."[26] Modern medical marvels are keeping us alive but at the price of experiencing a painstakingly long and gradual decline beset by pain, bedsores, and loss of function and cognition.

I hope for a "Niagara Falls" end of life, meaning that I hope to live fully to a ripe old age and then swiftly decline (plunge over the waterfall) and die a gentle, fast, and peaceful death. The chances of that happening are remote. It's much more likely I will slowly dwindle into increasing frailty and senility as my vital organs (or perhaps one in particular, like my heart) gradually fail. The irony of my open-heart surgery in 2021 at age seventy-three is that I may live a few years longer, but I still have to die of something that may be far more painful and lingering than a heart attack.[27]

I love life, and my support for right-to-die laws does not mean I don't want to live as long as possible. I would be delighted to live long and die naturally, provided any pain is well managed and my dignity, autonomy, and agency remain intact. But if I'm among those who suffer appallingly, I will gently hasten my death through MAID, VSED, terminal sedation, or other means. This is not an act of cowardice or escapism but an act of common sense and rationality. It makes no sense to live with an unacceptable quality of life when nothing of any value can be accomplished by doing so.

I would be hypocritical if I were to write this book but not do any of the planning I recommended on these pages. In appendix I, you can find examples of letters I have written to my family describing how I would like to be treated at the end of my life and how I hope to die. The most important thing I've done is to talk about my wishes with my wife, Gail, and my three daughters so they can represent me well if I cannot communicate with my doctors. I've also written several legacy letters or ethical wills, which you can find in appendix II. And appendix IV describes my wishes for my burial and memorial service.

I hope to approach my death with the same serenity as Isaac Asimov, the scientist and author. In his final book, *Asimov Laughs Again: More than 700 Favorite Jokes, Limericks, and Anecdotes*, he writes, "I'm afraid that my life has just about run its course and I really don't expect to live much longer . . . and I have no complaints."[28] He goes on, "In my life, I have had (my wife) and I have had my daughter and my son. I have had a large number of good friends. I have had my writing. . . . No matter what happens to me now, it's been a good life, and I am satisfied with it."

At some point, we each need to recognize that our life has been completed and accept that it is time to die. When this happens, hopefully we will be at home with a lucid mind and a clear conscience, enjoying the love and affection of loved ones, and focused on what matters most to us as we gently and peacefully slide toward death.

* * * * *

I hope this book has helped you accept your finitude, eventual physical oblivion, and death more calmly and serenely. I hope the knowledge that you will die will lead you to find more meaning and purpose in your life. Transiency does not make a blooming rose less precious. Our awareness that life is fleeting and temporary does not mean that our lives should be devoid of joy, value, and intention. The reverse is true. Awareness of our transience and the brevity of life can drive our desire to search for meaning and eschew ennui, languor, and purposelessness.

Pondering on death and dying motivates us to focus on designing and pursuing a life of giving, fulfillment, and purpose. Death makes us think about the meaning of our lives and the legacy we leave behind. I hope this book has been "an awakening experience" for you.[29] At some point, we'll all die. It's the debt we must pay for the amazing gift of existence. We'll live on in our family, friends, and loved ones. We'll live on in the society we helped shape, in the stories that will be told and retold about us, and in the lives of others we've inspired.

Death is a transformative teacher, but few want to become willing students. I hope this book encourages you to become a student of your own end of life and to determine what you can do to achieve a good death. I hope you have a spirited and robust old age, live as long as possible, agree only to treatments that align with your goals, and have total patient agency. When the time comes, I hope you have a rapid and brief deterioration and a painless death at home, surrounded by your loved ones. I hope you will be serene at the moment of your death and have no fear or anxiety.

Examples of Letters Describing End-of-Life Wishes

A Letter to My Family about My End-of-Life Wishes
Summary of Letter

I do not want my death to be protracted or lingering, especially if I am bed-bound and cognitively impaired. The quality of my life is more important to me than its length.

Highly intensive medical technology for older people is rarely helpful and often only causes suffering. I don't want to end up hooked to tubes and machines. I want to be home with my loved ones or in an inpatient hospice like Casey House if it is too challenging to take care of me at home.

As I enter the last phase of my life, the following are important to me: being able to talk with all of you, being mentally alert and competent, preserving my quality of life, having autonomy and independence, being comfortable and free of pain, leaving good memories for all of you, dying quickly to avoid wasteful and expensive care.

I love so much about my life—being active, spending time with grandkids, writing, giving talks, and volunteering—that, if none of these activities were possible for me to enjoy anymore, I would want to go out peacefully without a lot of heroics. I want my doctor to refer me to hospice as soon as I am eligible.

If I'm severely compromised (e.g., by dementia or other illness) and unlikely to regain my ability to recognize loved ones, I'd consider my life over and want you to carry out my wishes for a peaceful death. Please do not work to prolong my life.

I believe if I have an irreversible illness or intractable pain, I have the right to end my life in any way I choose—a right to death with dignity.

I support terminal sedation, medical aid in dying (MAID), and voluntarily stopping eating and drinking (VSED). I want access to MAID medications (if legal) so I have the option of taking a lethal dose of medicine. I do not want my life prolonged artificially after it has ceased to be the life I want.

End of Summary

The full letter now follows:

Dear Gail, Kim, Sujay, Tina, CJ, Jenny, and Chase,

Every day, I'm so grateful we are all alive and healthy, and I hope we stay that way for a very long time!

As you know, I feel strongly about the importance of discussing how we want to be treated at the end of our lives and how the time to have that discussion is sooner rather than later. As the old maxim goes, we should repair the roof when the sun is shining.

So, this letter is my way of getting the discussion started! My personal mission statement outlines my views on death and dying, and this letter supplements what I wrote there.

The nonprofit organization Compassion and Choices, as well as the outstanding books *Finish Strong: Putting Your Priorities First at Life's End*, by Barbara Coombs Lee, and *The Art of Dying Well: A Practical Guide to a Good End of Life*, by Katy Butler, have informed this letter, and I am grateful to them.

Health-Care Agents

Gail is my health-care agent (or proxy) and will speak for me if I cannot. If Gail dies before I do or is incapacitated and unable to act as my health-care agent, then Kim, Tina, and Jen will be my health-care agents.

One of my goals with this letter is to give you the confidence to make hard decisions on my behalf if you must. In giving you this confidence, I also hope to provide you with peace of mind because you will know that you honored my wishes and that whatever decisions you made had my blessing.

Valuing the Time We Have Left

You might be thinking, "Why do we have to think about all this morbid, gloomy stuff?" My answer is that I love being alive, and it is sad to think about life ending, but knowing my life will end and facing that fact forthrightly doesn't make me feel morbid or gloomy. Instead, it makes me value the time I have left and strengthens my determination to protect its quality.

We plan for vacations to get the most out of them. We plan for retirement. We plan for our children to attend college. We plan for all the important events and developments in our lives. And yet, when it comes to the end of our lives, we tend not to think or talk about it. I believe this is a mistake.

Many Older People Don't Get What They Want

Most people want to stay in their homes toward the end of their lives. They want as much independence as possible and to be surrounded by friends and family. They want gentle and meaningful interactions with loved ones and to be free of suffering and pain.

But that isn't what most people get because they haven't prepared and planned ahead of time. Too many people begin to consider these questions only when a health crisis hits, which is a terrible time to make crucial decisions, such as whether you want CPR, surgery, or mechanical ventilation.

What Is a Good Death?

One of my life goals is to usher all of you gently through the process of my death so that, in retrospect, it is a positive, memorable, and loving experience for you.

I don't want you to suffer by watching me suffer. I do not want to be seen and remembered in a sad, pitiful state. I want to die *before* becoming a stranger to you through the cruel ravages of old age, particularly if I become demented.

I want my death to be peaceful and gentle, but I also want my exit from this world to be a meaningful, memorable, and even sacred time for all of you. So many survivors are traumatized by what they witness as their loved one dies in an ICU, with doctors frantically attempting to keep the dying patient alive for another few hours or days. I don't want you to be traumatized by my death.

When I approach the end of my life, which may be many years away, I want to ensure that my values and preferences are respected and honored so that I can achieve a good death, one free of pain, suffering, regrets, unfinished projects, and ineffective medical treatments, and, at the same time, one full of love, peace, and gentleness.

I want to make the most of those last few weeks and months of my life and have the opportunity to say goodbye to each of you.

I aim to "walk through the valley of the shadow of death" with stoicism and courage, bringing cheer and comfort to those around me.

My Death

My healthy lifestyle (and major surgeries for prostate cancer and heart disease) decrease the chance of my premature death but increase the likelihood of death by a chronic and painful illness like congestive heart failure.

A slow death in this way is often terrible. A peaceful and gentle death requires a strategy or plan. Leaving it to chance will likely result in prolonged suffering and futile overmedicalization that only wastes money and depletes precious resources. I want us all to be able to talk about it. Dying should not be a taboo topic.

Mommy/Gail and I disagree about whether my mother's four years in a nursing home were what she would have desired. I am pained by the memories of her loss of functionality and dignity, and I am clear that I want to prevent what happened to her from happening to me.

I do not want my death to be protracted or lingering, especially if I am bed-bound and cognitively impaired. *The quality of my life is far more important to me than its length.*

My Motivation for Writing This Letter

In addition to letting you know my wishes for the end of my life, I hope this letter will help *you* achieve good deaths when your lives end, hopefully many years after I die.

My goal is to set an example of how to have a good death, and fulfilling this goal will imbue my life with meaning and purpose until my last breath.

I am conscious that how I die will set an example to all of you who come after me. I hope you will write a letter similar to this to your loved ones when you are still in the prime of your lives. It would supplement your advance directive—as this letter does mine.

We each need to spell out what we want so we have some control over what happens to us. Death is unavoidable and can happen at any time. Better to approach it intentionally than haphazardly.

Make Sure My Doctors Are Candid and Honest with Me

I have written the attached letter to my doctor telling him how I want to be treated. Still, for many reasons, doctors are often reluctant to tell their patients that cures will no longer work and that it's time for comfort care, hospice, and efforts to maintain a high quality of life as long as possible.

Please make sure my doctors are candid with you and me and tell all of us the truth about the effectiveness of additional treatments. I always want to know the truth about my condition, treatment options, and the effectiveness of treatments. I don't want to be deceived or misled.

Inflicting Overmedicalization on Older People

As long as I am thriving and vibrant, I welcome care that will restore my health and help me retain a high quality of life.

Knowing that highly intensive medical technology for people in their eighties and nineties often doesn't work and causes undue suffering, I don't want to end up hooked to tubes and machines. I don't want to be isolated in an ICU, confused, ventilated, intubated, and in pain. I want to be home with my loved ones (all of you!) or in an inpatient hospice like Casey House if it proves too challenging to take care of me at home.

I do not want to live as long as possible, regardless of my quality of life. If the prognosis is grave, my physical state is dire, and there is little chance that I will ever regain mental or physical function, I want to be allowed to die peacefully and as quickly as possible.

Being assigned to an ICU and hooked up to multiple machines would be worse than death for me. The pain, discomfort, isolation, lack of autonomy, and hopelessness would be unbearable and torturous.

At the end of my life, I do not want mechanical breathing and artificial ventilation, tracheotomy, CPR, artificial nutrition and hydration (through a nasogastric tube or a PEG tube), hospital intensive care, electroshocks to my heart, medications to stimulate heart function, dialysis, chemotherapy or radiation therapy, or surgery.

There may be other machines, drugs, or approaches yet to be invented that would, if used on my body at the end of life, add a few hours or days of diminished existence. Please know that I do not want any such "assistance."

Instead, I want the end of my life to be driven by quality-of-life issues and palliative care rather than invasive and painful medical care, especially if the prognosis is poor.

If a hospital or any health-care person associated with them or involved in my care intentionally ignores my advance directive and dementia coda and overmedicalizes me, contrary to my wishes, please take legal action against the institutions and the persons who disregarded my wishes so we can set a legal precedent (based on the "wrongful prolongation of life") that others in the future must respect and follow advance directives.

Lawsuits in Georgia, Alaska, and elsewhere have resulted in large monetary settlements and, more importantly, put everyone involved in health care on notice that they should pay attention to advance directives.

As I Enter the Last Phase of My Life

As I enter the last phase of my life, the following are important to me: being able to talk with all of you, being mentally alert and competent, preserving my quality of life, having autonomy and independence, being comfortable and free of pain, leaving good memories for all of you, dying quickly rather than lingering in agony, and avoiding wasteful and expensive care.

Each of you knows me and can see what brings me joy. Your observations and knowledge, combined with the information and directives in this letter and our conversations, will guide you to recognize the point at which a good death is better than a "heroic" medically produced life.

Dementia, medications, or my physical condition may make it hard for me to recognize when that point has arrived. I am counting on each of you to be attentive to the quality of my life, know what I value, and be courageous in making the decisions necessary to end my life with dignity.

I intend to have a disciplined routine to give my life structure up to the end. Even as I become frail, I plan to feel joy and gratitude and continue doing everything I love, like nurturing my grandchildren, volunteering, writing, reading, giving talks, seeing friends, drawing, juggling, and playing the piano.

As my world contracts and shrinks, I intend to be at peace with that reality. I will look at society and accept that I am departing from it and that it will carry on after my death with barely a flicker.

How to Treat Me at the End of My Life

Before I begin actively dying, I'd like lots of visitors and to be surrounded by Gail, my daughters, sons-in-law, grandchildren, and great-grandchildren. I want my loved ones to combine grieving with celebratory food, drink, music, stories, roasting, and toasting.

As I approach the end, I would love to hear you recall our happy times together and your fun and joyful memories. It would bring me enormous pleasure to talk to each of you, including my beloved and precious grandchildren, about the good times we have shared. If conversation is no longer possible for me, your presence, your words, and your love will bring me comfort.

I'd love to have photos of my loved ones (all of you!) in my room near my bed. Also, I would like to have my hand held and to be talked to when possible, even if I don't seem to respond to the touch and voice of others.

At the end of my life, I would like to be kept fresh and clean, and I would like my lips and mouth to be kept moist to stop dryness.

I'd love to die at home with hospice care, but I realize that, at some point, this may impose too big a burden on members of my family. If that is the case, then it's OK for me to spend my last days in Casey House, a beautiful inpatient facility with Montgomery Hospice (www.montgomeryhospice.org).

I want to be conscious and lucid enough to say goodbye as I die. But, on the other hand, I also welcome pain control and realize that painkillers may make me drowsy and non compos mentis. So, I am counting on you to help me juggle these two conflicting goals.

Please make sure that my doctors and nurses know about the kind of person I was before getting sick and senile. For example, show them a photo of me doing handstands in my seventies! And please protect me from well-meaning religious folk who want to convert me before I die.

I want my death to release love. I want you to celebrate my life, not mourn my death. My death is not a tragedy—at my age, no matter when death arrives, no one will say I died young!

I Want No Heroics

I love so much about my life—being active, spending quality time with grandkids, writing, giving talks, and volunteering—that, if none of that is possible, I want to go out peacefully without any medical heroics.

I want my doctor to refer me to hospice as soon as I am eligible. And if I'm in a hospital, I'd like a referral to palliative care at the earliest opportunity, even if I am undergoing curative treatment.

If it becomes clear that my remaining time is short no matter what treatments I receive, I'd like to do less instead of more. I do *not* want a tube put down my throat or inserted in my windpipe to keep me breathing. I do *not* want a PEG tube inserted into my stomach to feed me. Instead, I want a calm, gentle death.

If I'm severely compromised and unlikely to regain my ability to recognize loved ones, I consider my life over and want you to carry out my wishes for a peaceful death. If I have dementia and no longer recognize my beloved grandchildren, please do not work to prolong my life.

If I cannot respond to you with love and a sound mind, I ask you to collaborate with nature to see that my life ends as quickly as possible.

Please do not wait for advanced dementia, permanent unconsciousness, or terminal illness. An incapacitating stroke, an inability to move and think, stupor, delirium, or serious mental impairment should trigger the implementation of my exit strategy.

I see no purpose in prolonging my dying if it is painful, miserable, and hopeless. If I have lost all cognitive ability, I request that I *not* be spoon-fed.

I do not want my life prolonged by artificial means (medicines, machines, CPR, tube feedings, devices or techniques not yet invented, etc.) if I'm bedridden or cannot recognize and communicate with my family.

Seek Opportunities to Welcome Death's Approach

My life is full of loving, thinking, feeling, writing, talking, giving, teaching, volunteering, and laughing. If I cannot do those things and will never be able to do them, my life is over, and it's time for comfort care only.

If my mental function is seriously compromised with little chance for full recovery, please seek opportunities to encourage death's approach. Suppose, for example, I have pneumonia or another infection. Let my body go. Do not fight an infection with antibiotics if what remains after the drugs work is not worth fighting for. Are my kidneys faltering? Let them. Is my heart failing or my blood pressure falling? Do nothing. Am I refusing water and food? Good! Let it be.

Please look for what one expert in end-of-life issues, Dr. Joanne Lynn, calls "creative collaboration with the forces of nature." In other words, please take advantage of natural illnesses as they arise. Welcome my health failings as benefactors that have arrived to hasten my death. They should not be regarded as diseases to be attacked and combated with medical marvels.

I welcome aggressive treatment for pain and symptom relief while a disease takes its natural course, but artificially sustaining my life (that is, keeping me alive) while my quality of life drastically deteriorates would torment me unnecessarily.

If I Have Dementia

Advanced dementia is worse than death. I do not want to experience the end stages of dementia. I do not want to become seriously dysfunctional and very different from who I am today. Nor am I willing to experience substantially reduced mental function and an inability to talk and write.

Anything worse than mild cognitive decline is unacceptable to me and should trigger my exit strategy. I don't want the last years of my life to contradict all that went before, so I have added a dementia coda to my advance directive to underscore what I request in this letter.

If I have dementia, I am deeply concerned about the practical and emotional burdens this would put on those who love me and want to take care of me. Therefore, please remove all barriers to a natural, peaceful, and timely death. I want comfort care only. Please qualify me for hospice if you can.

Please make no attempt at resuscitation using CPR or any other method. Please ask my doctor to sign a do-not-resuscitate order.

Please do not authorize any treatment or procedure that might prolong or delay a natural death or prolong or increase my suffering. Do *not* intubate me. Do *not* give me intravenous fluids. Do *not* transport me to a hospital. Do *not* treat my infections with antibiotics, but give me painkillers instead. Please ask my medical team to deactivate all medical devices, such as defibrillators and pacemakers, that might delay my death.

Please do not coerce or even coax me to eat. If I'm eating, let me eat whatever I want. Do *not* allow a feeding tube for me. If one is inserted, please have it removed immediately. Please forbid dialysis. I want comfort care only, and I want to avoid all treatments that might be painful, agitating, or prolong my dying. Please give me opioids to relieve any pain. If I need to be institutionalized, please send me to an inpatient hospice like Casey House.

My Right to Die

I believe that, if I have an irreversible illness or intractable pain, I have the right to hasten the end of my life in any way I choose—a right to death with dignity. I want a good death if I can no longer enjoy a good life.

I support medical aid in dying (MAID) and want access to MAID medications (if legal) so I have the option of taking a lethal dose of medicine. I do not want my life prolonged artificially after it has ceased to be the life I want.

Pain Relief and Palliative Sedation

If I'm in pain, breathless, or agitated, I want those symptoms relieved quickly and vigorously with morphine, even if the treatment unintentionally advances the time of my death or even causes my death. It is more important to enhance my quality of life if I'm seriously ill, even if the treatment shortens my life.

With severe pain, intensely labored breathing (dyspnea), or agitation, I welcome palliative (terminal) sedation.

Voluntarily Stopping Eating and Drinking (VSED)

I will use VSED (voluntarily stopping eating and drinking) to die if necessary. When there is no hope for recovery, my life is near an end, and I am no longer enjoying being alive, and assuming MAID is unavailable, I will intentionally hasten my death using VSED. I will initiate VSED before I stop recognizing loved ones and cannot communicate. I believe that VSED is justified when the burdens of my life outweigh the benefits.

VSED causes death by dehydration within eight to fourteen days. Doctors say it is peaceful and causes little suffering *when adequately supported by good oral care and pain-relieving analgesics*. Its slowness also provides time for reflection, family interactions, and mourning.

I would rather end my life using VSED or MAID than suffer the despair of a lengthy stay trapped in an ICU on mechanical life support.

Because of the legality and availability of VSED, I don't think I will need to use the Swiss nonprofit Dignitas to end my life unless the hospice I'm using refuses to support me using VSED (or MAID if it becomes legal). However, I'm prepared to use Dignitas (or another similar Swiss nonprofit organization) if my other options for a peaceful exit are blocked.

I Plan to Obtain a DNR (Do-Not-Resuscitate) Order

When the time is right, I plan to obtain a DNR (do-not-resuscitate) order (i.e., no CPR) and a MOLST (Medical Orders for Life-Sustaining Treatment) from my doctor. DNR is also called DNAR (do not attempt resuscitation) or AND (allow natural death).

MOLST will support my advance directive. An advance directive is ostensibly a legal document, while a MOLST is a medical order. A MOLST provides a tool for patients near the end of life to control their medical treatment better than advance directives alone, though both are important.

Please remember what I wrote earlier: If a hospitalist (a hospital doctor) chooses to ignore my advance directive and gives me painful treatments even though I have explicitly said not to, please sue the doctor for medical malpractice and "wrongful prolongation of life."

Such a lawsuit would help future dying people be treated with more compassion and teach hospital administrations that there are severe consequences for failing to adhere to an advance directive.

A Brief Ceremony after I Die (If It Helps You)

I am indebted to author and science writer Katy Butler for the following idea. In many cultures, washing and anointing the body with oil after death is traditional. Katy Butler describes how nurses are now bringing a beautiful version of this ancient ceremony into hospital rooms.

This "bathing and honoring" practice may help loved ones say goodbye. A death doula could help facilitate it. Only do this ritual or ceremony if it is helpful to you. I'll be dead, so, at this point, all the focus is on all of you and what brings you comfort, solace, and peace.

OK, here is the ceremony: After I have died, perhaps my death doula or some of you might wash and dress my body (rather than letting my body be taken immediately to a funeral home). Then, if you felt like it, you could anoint my body with lavender oil using the following nurses' ceremony:

As my hair is anointed with fragrant oil, a family member recites, "We honor Chris's hair that the wind has played with." Next, a dab of oil is gently rubbed on my brow as another family member says, "We honor Chris's brow, the birthplace of his thoughts." "Chris" would be replaced by "Dad" or "Grandpa," as appropriate. Then, the ceremony would continue as follows, with each line said by someone in the room, and my name (Chris, Dad, Grandpa) would be inserted as appropriate in each succeeding sentence.

We honor your eyes that have looked on us with love and viewed the beauty of the earth.

We honor your nose, the gateway of breath.

We honor your ears that listened to our voices and concerns.

We honor your lips that have shared so much wisdom and knowledge.

We honor your shoulders that have borne burdens and strength.

We honor your heart that has deeply loved us.

We honor your arms that have embraced us and held us.

We honor your hands that have held our hands and done so many things in this life.

We honor your legs that carried you into new places and new challenges.

We honor your feet that forged your path through life.

We give thanks for the gifts you have given us in our lives.

We give thanks for the memories that we created together.

We have been honored to be a part of your life.

I will write separately about my legacy letter, obituary, memorial service, and how to dispose of my body.

Thanks for reading this letter and implementing it to the best of your ability.

Love,
Chris/Dad/Grandpa
XXXOOO

* * * * *

A LETTER TO MY DOCTOR
Dear Dr. Watkins,

It is important to me to have excellent and compassionate care and stay as healthy and active as possible throughout my life. Thank you for all you have done and will continue to do to preserve my health. When I approach the end of my life, I want treatment to alleviate suffering. Most importantly, I want to ensure that the experience can be peaceful for my family and me as death becomes imminent.

If measures are available that may extend my life, I would like to know their chances of success and their impact on the quality of my life. If I choose not to take those measures, I ask for your continued support, even if that choice goes against medical advice.

If my condition becomes incurable and death is the only predictable outcome, I would prefer not to suffer but would rather die in a humane and dignified manner. Therefore, I would like your assurance of the following:

1. You will tell me candidly and honestly when further treatments are futile.

2. If it becomes clear that my remaining time is short, regardless of treatment, I want you to do less instead of more.

3. If I can speak for myself, my wishes will be honored. If not, the requests from my wife, Gail, and my advance directive (which you have) will be honored.

4. You will make a referral to Montgomery Hospice as soon as I am eligible.

5. You will support me with all options for a gentle death. These include VSED, palliative sedation, and, if medical aid in dying is authorized in Maryland, providing a prescription for medications I can self-administer to help my death be peaceful and dignified.

I hope for your assurance that you will support my personal end-of-life care choices as listed above.

I am attaching a letter to my family that explains how I want to be treated at the end of my life.

I hope you will accept this statement as a fully considered decision expressing my deeply held views. If you feel unable to honor my requests, please let me know now so I can make choices about my care based on that knowledge. Thank you.

Very best,
Chris Palmer

* * * * *

A LETTER TO MY FAMILY ABOUT ENDING MY LIFE

(In Case I Ever Need It)

Drafted on December 7, 2022 (but the date on the final letter, if ever used, would be much later)

To my precious family and friends,

I have decided to end my life because of the continued pain and unbearable suffering from heart disease.

I have lived a full, complete, meaningful, and useful life, but I have had enough and no longer wish to continue.

I am a wreck and only a relic of the energetic, productive, and creative person I used to be.

I have taken advantage of all the available medical care and interventions. I have decided that further medical treatments are useless and will only hurt me and worsen my life.

This decision is mine alone. I am in a rational and calm state of mind and feel completely at ease with this decision. I am not depressed or mentally unstable.

No one has helped me with this decision to end my life, and no one, including the beneficiaries of my estate, has put pressure on me to do so.

I support the Final Exit Network (FEN) and believe in its mission. I have chosen to die now.

If I am discovered before I stop breathing, I forbid anyone, including doctors and paramedics, to attempt to resuscitate me. If I am revived against my wishes, I shall take legal action against anyone who helped in that action.

Please add the following language to my obituary:

Chris took his own life in a rational self-deliverance toward the end of a terminal disease relating to his heart. He did this not out of cowardice or escapism but because it made no sense to continue living subhumanly with an unacceptable quality of life when nothing good or loving or kind could be accomplished. He died with a heart full of love, gratitude, and appreciation for all those he loved and who had supported him in his life.

Thank you for your understanding.
Love, Chris/Dad/Grandpa
XXXOOO

Appendix II

Examples of Legacy Letters and Ethical Wills

To my precious family:

Dear Gail, Kimmie, Tina, Jenny, Sujay, CJ, Chase, Kareena, Neal, JJ, Max, Sammy, Aiden, Connor, and Kim's soon-to-be third baby,

If you are reading this, it means that I have died. Perhaps it will be suddenly and unexpectedly, or perhaps after a long illness, from something like prostate cancer.

I hope I had a chance to say goodbye to you all. If not, then this letter is designed to fill that sad omission.

For decades now, I've wrestled with the problem of how best to prepare Kimmie, Tina, and Jenny if I were to die suddenly. One worry was the thought that Mommy and I might perish together in, say, a plane crash. The chances are highly remote, but it could happen. Mommy and I periodically talk about it. As the years have passed, this has become less of a worry for us because you are all growing up and can take care of yourselves.

On October 12, 2006, I wrote the following letter, and whenever Mommy and I left home for a trip together, I placed it in the middle of my desk where it would be easily found. Mommy wrote a similar letter at about the same time, and I would always leave copies of both letters side-by-side on my desk. Okay, here is my October 12, 2006 letter (I would include Mommy's letter too, but she has no electronic copy of it):

Darling Precious Kimmie, Tina, and Jenny,

If you are reading this, something terrible has happened. Whatever happened, remember that you made Mommy and me the happiest people in the world. We couldn't have died feeling happier, more content, and more at peace.

We are incredibly proud of each of you. You are strong, loving, resourceful, beautiful, courageous, bold, reflective, tenacious, caring, determined, intelligent, and wise. You are living honorable and wonderful lives. The world is a better and richer place for you being here.

A few days ago, Mommy asked me, "What are you most proud of in your life?" Without hesitation, I said, "Kim, Tina, and Jenny." I also now add Sujay to that list.

You are all set to continue leading vibrant, optimistic, and energetic lives, bringing joy and love to all you come into contact with. Mommy and I know you will continue to live happy, rewarding, and fulfilling lives. We are the luckiest parents in the world and will always adore you.

Remember, we will be at all the big events in your lives in the same way Sujay's father and my parents were at Kim's wedding.

Please tell your children my biggest sadness is not having the opportunity to be a loving, mischievous, and wise grandfather.

I love you more than I can say.

Your loving dad,

XXXOOO

As I say, if you are reading this letter, it means that I have died. This letter (the one you are holding) is designed to update the one above from 2006. I have found inspiration from the Stanford Life Review project. Here is another useful link.

If you are experiencing grief and sadness, I hope you'll be okay. Grief is exacerbated by regrets, but I hope we've all lived in a way together that any regrets are insignificant or very minor.

A companion letter to this is my January 9, 2019 letter (which I sometimes call a legacy or heirloom letter) describing the nonfinancial family assets Mommy and I are leaving you. That January 9, 2019 letter is tied to the shared Google Drive that contains many family documents, including letters, eulogies, mission statements, journals, books, family history, stories, etc.

I want to tell you how incredibly grateful I am to all of you for being the family that many husbands and fathers only dream about. I've been extraordinarily lucky, especially meeting and falling in love with Gail in 1972. You have all been so loving, so caring, so thoughtful, so generous, and so affectionate.

I am so proud of all of you:

1. Gail, for being such a loving, amazing, compassionate, and understanding wife, life partner, and mother;

2. Kim, for being such a loving and capable mom, wife, and professional, for all the books you've written helping people, and for being a wonderful daughter;

3. Tina, for being such a loving and competent mom, wife, and professional, for all the patients you've helped as a family doctor, and for being a wonderful daughter;

4. Jenny, for being such a loving wife and capable lawyer, for all the pro bono clients you've helped, and for being a wonderful daughter;

5. Sujay, for your love of reading (especially history!), your equanimity, your outstanding fathering, and your love and caring for Gail and me;

6. CJ, for your endless curiosity and love of learning, for your outstanding fathering, and the way you always make Gail and me feel so welcome when we visit you and Tina;

7. Chase, for getting your job at Google, for your determination to succeed, and for the touching way you talked to Gail and me about your desire to marry Jenny;

8. Kareena, Neal, JJ, Max, Sammy, Aiden, Connor, and Kim's about-to-be-born baby, for the indescribable joy you bring me, your love of games and play, your wonderful questions, and your inexhaustible love of learning.

Remember the vacation we all spent together in Monterey in August 2017? How much fun was that?! Here is an email I sent you all afterward with some of our memories:

1. Surfing (Kim, Sujay, CJ, and Chase)

2. Swimming in Jen and Chase's pool with JJ

3. Whales lunge feeding and tail slapping

4. Anchovies jumping out of the ocean onto the beach in countless numbers

5. Birds flying in lyrical and lithe murmurations

6. Beach fire on the beach and fire pit

7. Reading the *Circus Ship* book to the grandkids

8. Train ride through the redwoods

9. Visit the Monterey Aquarium

10. JJ playing tennis

11. Max's funny "old man" expressions

12. Neal doing exercises

13. Kareena showing how she can do two dances at the same time

14. Gift of a special book from JJ for my 70th birthday

15. Talking to K and N on the beach

16. Sujay's 40th birthday and my 70th

17. Watching Wimbledon-level tennis at the Nordic Natural Challenger

18. Playing tennis with CJ

19. Watching Tina and CJ play tennis

20. Tina and I having a handstand competition

21. Happy Hour every day at 5 pm in our hotel room

22. Kim's branding: "Cousin Time"

23. Hide and seek with K, N, and JJ

24. Playing diving games in the pool at Dinah's with Kareena and Sujay

25. Planning for Jen and Chase's December 9 wedding

26. Kim and Sujay enjoying the Carmal Refuge water resort

27. Gail arranging everything (thank you, my love!)

28. Feeding ducks and fish at Dinah's

29. Neal and JJ holding hands as they walked together to the train station

30. JJ's 3rd birthday party, all the neighbors and the piñata, plus the train ride

31. Seeing Mark and his five kids

32. Going to Menlo Church with Tina, CJ, JJ, and Max for the evening service

33. Two dinners at Tina and CJ's

34. Babysitting K and N while the other grownups had a drink

35. "Ceej" and "Suj" joke

36. Talk of moving to Denver

37. Having Kareena, Neal, JJ, and Max spend time together

38. Having Kim, Tina, and Jen spend time together (as well as Sujay, CJ, and Chase)

39. Spike ball (thanks to Jen and Chase)

40. Chase and I agreeing that kids need moral education

41. Getting all of us together and realizing these times are special

42. Chase's top secret, and still secret, Fitbit project

43. Jenny trying on her wedding dress and having it sent back to China

44. Chase giving me sangrias

45. Max in the process of learning to walk

46. Giving JJ and Max baths (and Gail washing their hair with no tears)

47. Dinner with Jen on the last night

48. Dinners at Sanderlings

49. Getting rides on golf carts to get to and from the beach

50. Tina and CJ playing golf

51. Kareena and Neal showing JJ the red thimble magic trick

52. Kids playing Geronimo with me

53. Seeing Chance

54. Playing catch with a tennis ball on the beach.

I have so many happy and meaningful memories from my life. Here are just a small handful:

- Gail: dancing lessons, playing tennis, club parties, watching *The Crown*, StoryWorth questions
- Kim: when your first book was published
- Tina: when you finished your medical training
- Jenny: the trip you took with Mommy after taking the bar exam
- Sujay: sharing history books on tape
- CJ: playing tennis
- Chase: your personal training sessions
- Kareena: Admiral of the Fleet
- Neal: Geronimo
- JJ: the book you wrote for me for my seventieth birthday
- Max: your smile
- Sammy, Aiden, Connor, and Kim's about-to-be-born baby: I was so looking forward to getting to know you

Thank you to all of you for everything you have done for me. I have so much to thank you each for, including the following:

- Gail: for your profound love, your wisdom, your values, your empathy, and for teaching me so much
- Kim, Tina, and Jenny: for being fantastic daughters—so loving, so loyal, so affectionate, so generous, so capable, so wise—I learned so much from each of you
- Sujay, CJ, and Chase: for being fantastic sons-in-law—you are the sons I never had

- Kareena, Neal, JJ, Max, Sammy, Aiden, Connor, and Kim's about-to-be-born baby: for letting me be the playful, loving grandpa I always dreamed of being

I want you all to know that I love you very much.

- Gail: I love you for being the most beautiful and wonderful wife a man could ever have
- Kim, Tina, and Jenny: I love you for being incredible daughters
- Sujay, CJ, and Chase: I love you for being the best husbands Kim, Tina, and Jenny could ever marry
- Kareena, Neal, JJ, Max, Sammy, Aiden, Connor, and Kim's about-to-be-born baby: I love you for being the most spectacular grandchildren a grandpa could ever wish for

Thank you all for everything you have done for me. It has been an extraordinary honor to have been a part of your lives. I know you'll find peace, love, and joy in the years to come.

I want to end with a few specific goodbye messages:
- Gail, my love: do marry again if you'd like to!
- Kim, Tina, and Jenny: take care of each other and of Mommy— never let anything come between you
- Sujay, CJ, and Chase: thanks for taking care of Kim, Tina, and Jenny and for loving them so profoundly
- Kareena, Neal, JJ, Max, Sammy, Aiden, Connor, and Kim's about-to-be-born baby: I know you'll grow up to be strong, loving, successful, fulfilled, and resilient, that you'll bring joy and light to all those you connect with, and that you'll each leave a special and precious legacy that you can be proud of

I love you.

Chris/Dad/Grandpa

XXXOOO

****

Darling Kimmie, Tina, and Jenny,

As you know, I'm writing a book on death and dying, and one thing I've learned is that postponing important talks until one is on one's deathbed is a big mistake. Deathbed conversations are rarely rewarding. Everyone is grieving, and the person dying is usually barely conscious, frail, cognitively impaired, and maybe in pain and discomfort.

So, I want to tell you now how much I love you and not put it off to a time when I may have trouble speaking and thinking. I'm at the peak of good health, so now is the perfect time for this letter.

This letter supplements my five-page January 11, 2019, letter I sent to the whole family, which I call my "goodbye" or "gratitude" letter, and my June 20, 2020, letter to the three of you, expressing why I am so proud of you.

This letter is also part of my ongoing project to write "toast letters" to family members and friends to let them know I love them. You are, of course, at the top of the list (along with Mommy) to receive a "toast" letter from me.

So, Kimmie, Tina, and Jenny, this is a toast to you!!!

I am so proud of you and so proud to be your father. You have helped make me supremely happy and content. You are thoughtful, generous, and affectionate while also having grit and tenacity.

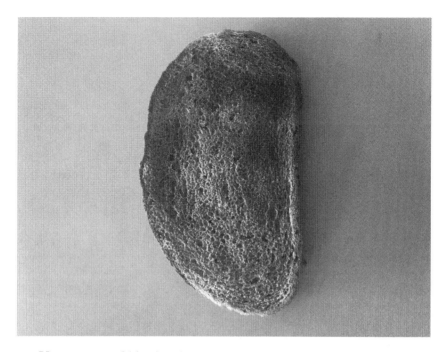

You are incredible daughters, and you are living honorable lives. I know the days seem long and exhausting. Your jobs are challenging (in a good way), kids have bad moods and tantrums, the laundry is relentless, and cleaning up constant messes is tedious—but the bigger picture is that you are living outstanding lives, and the world is richer in so many ways for you being here.

Mommy and I adore you and always will, even after we are gone. Thank you for bringing us so much joy. You are each so strong, resourceful, loving, capable, wise, and beautiful.

Not only are you competent and loving mothers, but you are also highly accomplished professionals. You've worked diligently to establish yourselves in challenging and esteemed career paths. Your peers, colleagues, and supervisors have a high regard for you.

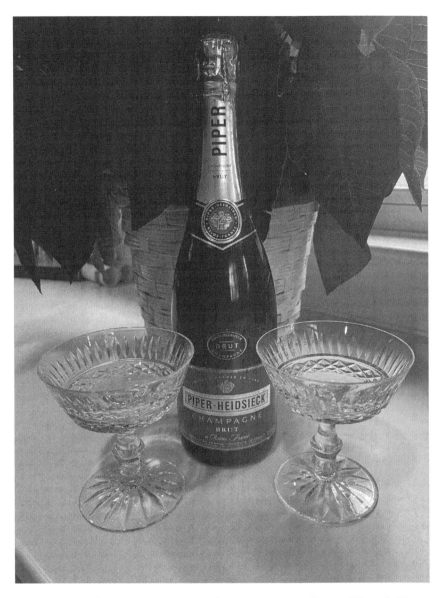

On top of all that, you married amazing men. Sujay, CJ, and Chase are the beloved sons Mommy and I never had. Mommy and I are as proud of them as we could be.

And then there are your children! Were grandparents ever blessed with a more adorable brood than our nine?! Kareena, Neal, JJ, Max, Sammy, Aiden, Connor, Dylan, and Charlie are wonderful, and they are wonderful in large part because they have stellar parents.

Your kids are flourishing because you create environments that encourage them to flourish. You—and your husbands—work hard to be the best parents possible.

You also do something that many parents neglect. Although you constantly have to make sacrifices for your family, you make an effort to take care of yourselves. You eat well, exercise whenever you can, and sleep as much as you can. (Sorry, Kimmie, I know Dylan is up half the night at the moment, so a good sleep for you is impossible.)

Good for you for doing your best to take care of yourselves. You can't take care of others if you are not healthy yourself, although I know how hard that is when you have babies and toddlers under your feet all the time.

Here are three stories about you that stick vividly in my mind:

1. Kimmie: When you were at Amherst, you realized in the first year or so that you were not making the quality friends you yearned for. You found yourself surrounded by mediocre, average people who weren't worthy of you. So, you were proactive in solving that problem. You looked around, saw Alison, realized she was exceptional, and went out of your way to befriend her. Because you took that initiative, you now have a special group of lifelong friends (KEPAC) from your college days. Writing this recalls fond memories of your college-era journalism—essays about coming home for Thanksgiving freshman year and your appreciation for my graduate gift journal.

2. Tina: The strength and grit you showed to survive the hardships of medical school and residency amaze me. When you were at UCSF, you sometimes had to get up at 4 a.m. and cycle in the dark and rain

through deserted streets to get to the hospital. You showed a lot of toughness, determination, and self-discipline to get through those hard times. I am also in awe of your ability to learn all the science you had to learn, especially biology and chemistry, to get through med school. That took a lot of admirable hard work and focus. Your experiences with street kids in Costa Rica, the homeless in India, and the TB wards in Botswana are other examples of times you showed your resilience and strength.

3. Jenny: The story I will select about you is your pregnancy with Aiden and Connor. When you learned you were having twins, you resolved that caring for those babies was your highest priority. You did everything possible to ensure that Aiden and Connor got off to the best possible start in life. Being pregnant with twins is arduous and exhausting, and you dealt with all the discomfort and physical awkwardness with poise, resilience, focus, and strength. You proactively took the best care of yourself when work demands might have tempted you to put work first—and you made it all the way to week thirty-seven! After Aiden and Connor were born, you took extra care to study up and hire help to get you through the early months. Writing all this reminds me that you always set goals and worked hard to achieve them, and, in doing that, you often took bold and courageous steps, like when you moved to SF, where you knew no one, to work for Brattle.

Those stories say a lot about your characters. You set high standards for yourselves, took on challenging and complex goals, and then planned your time effectively to accomplish those goals.

As you know, I've been collecting stories about you since you were born. And, as you also know, I've collected them into a fifty-page book called *Family Stories*. Of all the books and journals I've written relating to our family, that precious little book is one of my favorites.

You each got into the very top colleges in the country (Amherst, Dartmouth, Princeton) and thrived and blossomed there, and then went on to get accepted at top graduate schools (Chicago, UPenn, and Stanford), each of you with offers of substantial scholarships.

Of course, before college, you had all done exceedingly well at Holton-Arms and accepted early admission to your first-choice college.

You will each leave a significant mark on the world, and who knows what the future might hold for you. Here are a few possibilities:

- Writing books (or more books!)
- Making films
- Starting nonprofits
- Lavishing love on grandchildren and great-grandchildren
- Making new friends
- Writing letters to newspapers
- Pursuing exciting job and career opportunities
- Teaching
- Playing competitive tennis
- Running for public office
- Devoting yourselves to worthy volunteer responsibilities
- Pursuing minimalism
- Starting a newsletter or podcast
- Spreading joy and inspiration to all those you encounter
- Helping your families flourish and thrive
- Serving on the board of a nonprofit

When you get to my age, you might do what I've done and pursue new interests like juggling, drawing, playing the piano and singing, running a death-and-dying group, playing tennis, and being a hospice volunteer. All three of you are very good at challenging yourselves and constantly growing and learning. It's good always to be doing something hard.

One of my top goals in life has been to be the best possible father to you and to give you constant love, support, encouragement, and inspiration. I poured a lot of effort into learning how to parent because, unlike Mommy, I knew very little about it when Mommy and I got married. I had a lot to learn. Of course, I stumbled many times and made mistakes, but I was always amazed at how forgiving you were and how my mistakes never diminished your immense love for me.

Parenting you three girls gave my life incredible meaning and purpose. Nothing else came close to it, including my environmental work with films or my book writing. My overpowering love for you and intense feelings of responsibility for you made me into a new and better person with stronger values and a steadfast sense of purpose.

I'm deeply grateful to you, not only for the love you have for Mommy and me but also for the love you have for each other. You care about each other and are each other's best friends. Your relationship with each other is filled with respect, laughter, fun, enjoyment, and shared values.

You are so important to me. I treasure you each. Mommy and I are incredibly proud of you, and we love you more than words can convey.

Love, Dad

XXXOOO

* * * * *

To my three precious daughters, Kimmie, Tina, and Jenny,

Darling Kimmie, Tina, and Jenny,

I recently came across a six-minute video in which ten fathers and their (mostly) grown children were videotaped in pairs as the child asked the father, "What about me makes you proud?"

I found the video so moving and poignant that I sent it to my aging, death, and dying group in my most recent weekly letter to them.

Then, an idea occurred to me. I want to answer that question for you, and what better day to do that than Father's Day? Also, I don't want to wait to do this until I become frail and cognitively impaired from old age, and it's too late!

At first, I started drafting individual letters to each of you, but they were so overlapping that I decided it would be better to write the letter to all three of you.

Here you go:

Darling Kimmie, Tina, and Jenny,

I am proud of you for so many reasons that I don't know where to begin.

For a start, you are all such accomplished professionals. You've worked incredibly hard to establish yourselves in particularly challenging and competitive careers. I'm proud of you for doing so well and for being highly regarded by your colleagues, bosses, and subordinates.

I'm even prouder of you for what you've accomplished in your personal lives. You've each married a fantastic man. Sujay, CJ, and Chase are beloved sons-in-law, and Mommy and I are so proud and happy that they are now part of our family.

And your children! Wow! Where to begin?! I'm proud of you for being extraordinary mothers. I know it's not always easy. Raising kids is one of the most vexing jobs in the world and one of the most important.

Children can be exhausting, and being a mom often involves tedious work—now (during the pandemic) more than ever.

I'm proud of you for taking on the job of raising kids with dedication, devotion, and love. All three of you have incredible families, and Mommy and I are so grateful for all the love and affection we receive from you and your families.

Your families are flourishing because of the love and caring you (and your husbands) bring to the job of being the best parents you can be. You all have beautiful homes too!

I'm proud of you for taking care of yourselves, for eating healthily, for keeping fit, and for getting as much sleep as you can (which I know is not nearly enough).

I'm proud of you for the characters you have forged and the values you uphold. You are loving, wise, kind, patient, persevering, tough, resilient, determined, compassionate, and generous. You were a joy to raise.

Your sense of humor, your zest for life, your decency, your loving natures, your grit, your love of learning, and your capacity for friendship are all things that make me proud of you.

I'm proud of you for being *you*. Thank you for bringing Mommy and me so much profound joy. I'm proud of what you are making of your lives despite the hardships and setbacks that life brings to us all.

Some of my favorite recent highlights follow:

- Kimmie: How you give Kareena and Neal life challenges and other challenges during the Covid-19 shutdown—and the respect and warmth the NBC *Today Show* hosts show you (and how outstanding you are on TV)

- Tina: The love and values you bring to your loving documentation of your rich family life in your family blog—and the courage and strength of character you showed in your bold move to Colorado
- Jenny: The rave assessments you received recently during your annual review from the partners at your law firm—and the courage, resilience, and sound values you demonstrated during your challenging twin pregnancy

I love you—and thanks for blessing my life.

Yer ol' dad

XXXOOO

Appendix III

Example of a Eulogy

Eulogy for Jon Palmer

October 18, 2022

I'm Chris Palmer, Jon's twin brother, and I'm married to Gail, sitting over there. We're here from America.

Many of you know my twin brother as Jonny, but I called him Jon. Jon and I talked every Saturday morning. We had a special bond.

When we were toddlers, my mother said Jon and I had our own language that we could understand, but nobody else could. We shared a closeness during our childhood, doing everything together. We both had a built-in protector and best friend.

Our lifelong bond means his death is a terrible loss for me. Jon was a cherished part of my life.

Jon lived in the moment and didn't dwell on the future, something that people like me, who arguably spend too much time worrying about the future, can learn from. He was at ease with who he was, and he liked the person he was.

He had a straightforward philosophy of life and did not need or want very much. He wasn't into consumerism, and he wasn't greedy or pretentious. Instead, he enjoyed the simple things in life: friends, food, reading, socializing, dancing, cricket, and Bath rugby home games.

He didn't believe in overthinking things. He believed in "getting on with it," working hard, and focusing on what was in front of him. He loved playing sports back in the day and was a key figure in the local cricket team. And, yes, he loved his routines!

We gather today to celebrate Jon's life and mourn his unexpected death. He was taken from us too soon.

The poet Maya Angelou wrote,

When great trees fall, rocks on distant hills shudder,

Lions hunker down in tall grasses,

and even elephants lumber after safety.

Jon was like a great tree. He was always there. Always ready to help if you needed support. Always prepared to give advice and get you out of trouble. He was rock solid, trustworthy, and reliable.

His death is like a great tree falling.

There are three attributes of Jon I want to describe. **First,** how he always had your back. **Second,** how he was a devoted father to Hannah and Ross. And, **third,** how he was a good friend to so many and loved by so many.

First, he always had your back. He was always there for you. People in trouble gravitated toward him like boats hurrying to get to a safe harbor in a storm.

When we were young teenagers at boarding school at Dulwich College in London, Jon heard rumors that I would be the target of a physical attack by some senior boys. We were in different houses, and he took a considerable risk to reach me immediately to warn me. Jon had my back.

And he was always there, too, for our older brothers Timothy and Jeremy.

At Dulwich College, by the way, Jeremy was known as Palmer I, Tim as Palmer II, Jon as Palmer III, and I as Palmer IV.

My daughter Kimberly was about twenty years old and studying in London. She got a job at a grocery store, but the store managers were abusive. Kimberly told Jon about it, and he immediately fired off a stern letter threatening legal action unless they stopped their abuse. Jon had Kimberly's back.

Ross thinks that Jon having people's backs was a key part of what he enjoyed about being a criminal defense lawyer. People came to him for help, and he was immediately galvanized by that. As a result, he had a long, happy, and distinguished career at Withy King as a highly respected criminal and family lawyer, and he was instrumental in establishing and growing these departments in the firm.

Jon was also a great comfort to my parents as they became older. He was their only son in Bath, and they came to rely on him for support.

Jon, Hannah, and Ross had the following routine every Sunday: They would go for a game of pool and listen to the jukebox in the local pub, then go to my parents' house at 89 Bloomfield Avenue for lunch. After lunch, Jon often mowed my parents' lawn and trimmed the hedges. Jon had my parents' back.

Lisa told me that, before she and Jon were married, they climbed Snowdon one winter when the snow was deep. Unfortunately, they lost their way and crossed a steep slope with a massive drop. Here is how Lisa described what happened next:

> We had to dig our feet into the snow and lean out from the mountain because if you hugged the mountain, you would slide and most probably die. I froze with fear and didn't want to move, but Jon patiently and reassuringly got me to move—one step at a time. Jon didn't like the situation any more than I did and was putting himself at risk by helping me. Jon talked about this as the occasion he saved my life, and I think he did.

Jon was like a great tree, always there for family members who needed support.

The second attribute I want to highlight is that Jon was a devoted father to Hannah and Ross. He was so proud of them. He loved them dearly and would do anything for them. As a result, the three of them had a wonderful bond.

Ross told me that Jon had a strong sense of duty, which tended to be the language by which he communicated love and affection. Ross told me he was not very emotionally communicative, but he was always there for you. Caring for others, in his own way, was a core part of who Jon was.

Hannah and Ross told me Jon had quite a traditional approach to fatherhood. He wouldn't necessarily freely offer support—he would expect you to come to him and ask. But if you did and needed help, he would always give it. His main concern was that his children had the essentials. So he'd ask them, "Are you keeping healthy? Are you getting enough sleep? Are you living within your means?" And so on.

Ross told me the following:

> Dad did so many things for me over the years, including several trips to London when I was moving flats, taking us on countless holidays and outings. But I think a lot of it was the small things and always being

there when you needed him, if it was needing a lift, needing somewhere to stay, advice, and so on. He was a strong and stabilizing figure; he always checked up on us, ensured we had everything we needed, offered guidance, and arranged regular dinners, lunches, and coffees with us. He was a consistent, caring, and supportive figure, and for that I will always be grateful.

For Hannah and Ross, Jon was like a great tree, always there for them.

And the third attribute: Jon was a good friend and excellent company, something everyone here today can attest to. As Ross said to me recently, he was loved by so many.

A day or two after Jon died, I received an email from his long-term, close friend John Brownrigg lamenting Jon's death. John Brownrigg wrote,

> What a character! What a friend! His personality will always shine in my heart. I always felt he had my back and never doubted his friendship and support. He never failed to amuse and entertain and gave off warmth and humorous affection in spades. He was such an influence on my life, someone I was truly privileged to know.

Jon was smart and knowledgeable and could offer insights and perceptive comments on almost any topic.

He had a lovely capacity for friendship and was invariably upbeat and optimistic, an underrated character trait in the world. People like Jon, who bring a smile into the world, are precious. They help to lift us all up. Jon's cheerfulness was a gift in itself.

Jon was a friend to a wide network of people—from all walks of life. Ross told me,

> I can't count the times I would be out with Dad, and someone would come up to him and say thank you. I would ask Dad who that was, and

it was often someone who had gotten into trouble with the law. He did like the everyman.

Perhaps that came from his jobs as a student, selling ice cream, being a bus conductor, and being a waiter, where he interacted with a broad diversity of people.

Jon had a great sense of fun. During one winter vacation in our early thirties on an icy moor in Devon, we decided to go horse riding even though we barely knew how to ride. Assuming the horses would be docile and sluggish, we told the farmhands we knew how to ride, not realizing that the horses were itching for a fast gallop. We mounted the horses, they took off at breakneck speed, and we hung on for dear life. After a scary five-minute crazy gallop, the horses suddenly stopped, and we were thrown sprawling to the ground. Miraculously, we escaped serious injury.

And Jon was funny. I remember my father telling me when I was about twelve years old that Jon was good at making people laugh, and my father was right. My middle daughter Christina told me last week that whenever she thinks about Uncle Jon, she thinks about him laughing or making other people laugh.

To his many friends, Jon was like a great tree, always there for them.

Jon has died, but he will live on in our memories and our hearts.

He was a great father, grandfather, brother, twin, brother-in-law, cousin, friend, uncle, and solicitor. We will miss his sense of humor, his steadfastness, his strength, his practical wisdom, and his optimism.

Jon, thanks for being like a great tree. You were always there for us. We will not forget you.

I'll think of you every Saturday morning when we talk on the phone.

I'll think of you when I have a cup of tea and a good laugh.

I'll think of you when I see the one-inch scar on my right thigh, a memento from our roughhousing with a penknife when we were eleven.

And I'll think of you when I play with my twin grandsons: Jenny's Aiden and Connor. They are just like you and me.

I'll miss you, Jon. I know I never said this, but I want to say it now—I love you.

My twin brother Jon died at his home in Bath, England, on September 22, 2022. He was seventy-five.

APPENDIX IV

Example of a Letter Describing a Burial and Memorial Service

NOVEMBER 2, 2023

I'm drafting these notes to help my family (Gail, Kim, Sujay, Tina, CJ, Jenny, and Chase), and to ease the burden on them when I die.

I want a simple green burial at Reflection Park (attended by family and close friends), buried next to Gail. Pumphrey Funeral Home (301-652-2200) can transfer my body to Reflection Park and help with the death certificate. (Will Pumphrey, the CEO, is a friend.) Pumphrey's can refrigerate my body for a few days or even longer while you make the arrangements. No embalming!

The contact at Reflection Park is Dr. Basil Eldadah: eldadahb@gmail.com. Basil and I are friends. The address is 16621 New Hampshire Avenue, Silver Spring, Maryland. The phone number is 443-840-6775. The website is reflectionpark.org.

At Reflection Park, I recommend a simple commitment service in line with a "home funeral" or "community-led death care." Basil or Will Pumphrey can recommend a "home funeral guide" to help you with the arrangements if you need help. Basil and Will will happily help you in any way they can.

I want family members to be the pallbearers. Everyone would say something. Bring flowers to say goodbye. Take your time. Feel free to draw on my biodegradable casket and write messages on it.

I can imagine our daughters, grandchildren, and great-grandchildren visiting and talking to us in Reflection Park. It is a beautiful natural area of forty acres, bursting with trees, wildflowers, and nature. A green burial at Reflection Park seems particularly fitting since I devoted my professional life to conservation.

* * * * *

My thoughts below are for a memorial service (perhaps about an hour long), but they could easily be used (with appropriate adjustments) for a "living wake" or "living funeral" (a celebration of the life of a dying person held *before* the person dies when she can appreciate what is said).

I strongly favor living wakes. If you do a living wake with a large group of family and friends, there may be no need for a memorial service, but a living wake would likely only involve a small group (the family and a few friends).

The green burial at Reflection Park would be followed one or two months later by a memorial service or life celebration, loosely in line with the notes below.

Of course, you may prefer that the memorial service follow the green burial within a day or so. That would help Jenny and Tina because they would only have to make one trip to Bethesda, but it also means there is much work to do quickly. (The estate would pay for travel expenses.)

Venue: I recommend the Edgemoor Club (or Woodend). After the memorial service, there can be a catered party or reception for everyone at the same venue (paid for by the estate).

Whom to invite: Everyone who knows me well. See the list of my friends on pages 8 and 9 of my Personal Mission Statement. Friends in the Bethesda Metro Area Village, Montgomery Hospice, MacGillivray Freeman, the Office of Cemetery Oversight, the Funeral Consumers Alliance of Maryland & Environs, and the Edgemoor Club. And, of course, all our friends, neighbors, and tennis partners.

Officiant or funeral celebrant: The officiant or celebrant could be Gail, Kim, Tina, Jenny, Sujay, CJ, Chase, or whomever Gail designates. A fallback (if no one wants to do it!) is to hire a secular humanist celebrant from the Washington Ethical Society. I prefer having Gail, Kim, Tina, or Jenny be the celebrant. Their job is to keep the event on track and well orchestrated.

Starting the event: The celebrant might begin by reading aloud the following message from me to set the intention:

Hi everyone, thank you for coming today! My life was full and happy, and I have much to be grateful for. My death, though sad, is not a tragedy. I don't want this celebration of my life to be too solemn. Please remember the wonderful times we had together. Please share your stories and memories with my grandchildren to help them remember me. I hope to live on in the hearts I leave behind.

Eulogists: Kim, Tina, Jenny, grandchildren, friends, and anybody else who would like to speak. I would be honored if my family, including grandchildren, spoke. Gail may prefer not to speak.

Postcards for written stories: Ask everyone to write their memories and stories about me on postcards and send them to Gail so she can share them with our grandkids. If this is done before the memorial service, some of them could be read aloud at the memorial service for everyone to enjoy. Everyone would be given, either before the memorial service or as they arrive, a postcard with the prompt: "A favorite memory of Chris was . . .."

Program: This printed document can include one or more photos of me, a short bio, the program elements, a list of eulogists, etc. Perhaps add a "thank you" from the family to everyone for coming. The memorial service might look like this:

- Music as people enter (see below for music selections #1 through #5)
- Welcome from celebrant
- Message from me (see above)
- Eulogies from Kim, Tina, and Jenny (or perhaps one of them speaking on behalf of all of them)
- Reading #1 (see below)
- Eulogies from grandchildren (or maybe a few of them speaking on behalf of all of them)
- Music: "You Raise Me Up" by Josh Groban
- Eulogies from friends (if offered)

- Reading #2 (see below)
- Opportunity for others to speak
- Reading #3 (see below)
- A thank you for coming and an announcement that a reception will follow
- Music as people exit (see below for music selections #6 through #8)

Readings: I've selected three readings to be read by family members (or friends), and I have included them at the end of this memo for ease of reference:

1. "We Remember Them" by Sylvan Kamens and Rabbi Jack Riemer

2. "Our Lives Matter" by M. Maureen Killoran

3. "The Wolf Credo"

Music: I've listed below music that I like. The first few choices can be played as the memorial service starts (as people come in) and when it ends (as people exit). *Note*: This list of thirty-eight pieces can also be my playlist as I near death.

1. "I Did It My Way" by Frank Sinatra

2. "What a Wonderful World" by Louis Armstrong

3. "Go Down Moses" by Louis Armstrong

4. "Imagine" by John Lennon

5. "No Hard Feelings" by the Avett Brothers (CJ)

6. "Eleanor Rigby" by the Beatles

7. "Auld Lang Syne," sung by the Choral Scholars of University College Dublin

8. "Yesterday" by the Beatles

9. "Pie Jesu" by Charlotte Church (*Voice of an Angel*)

10. *Gymnopedie No. 1* by Erik Satie

11. *Gnossienne 1* by Erik Satie (played by Alessio Nanni)

12. "That's Alright" by Elvis Presley

13. "I Will Always Love You" (from *The Bodyguard*), by Whitney Houston

14. "Summertime" by Charlotte Church

15. "How Do" by Mary Chapin Carpenter

16. The music to *Downton Abbey*

17. "You Raise Me Up" by Josh Groban

18. "Like a Rolling Stone" by Bob Dylan

19. "You've Got a Friend" by James Taylor

20. "Bridge over Troubled Water" by Simon and Garfunkel

21. "Beat It," and "Thriller" by Michael Jackson

22. "Johnny B. Goode" by Chuck Berry

23. "For a Dancer" by Jackson Browne

24. "If I Can Help Somebody" by Mahalia Jackson

25. "Dance Me to the End of Love" by Leonard Cohen

26. "Breathe" by the Kennedys

27. "Wind beneath My Wings" by Bette Midler or Celine Dion

28. "Somewhere My Love (Lara's Theme)" from *Dr. Zhivago*

29. "Hallelujah" by Lucy Brown (Leonard Cohen)

30. "My Heart Will Go On" (from *Titanic*)

31. "I Will Remember You" by Sarah McLachlan

32. "The Way We Were" by Barbara Streisand

33. "Happy" by Pheral Williams

34. "Down at the Twist N Shout" by Mary Chapin Carpenter

35. "Can't Stop the Feeling (Sunshine in My Pocket)" by Justin Timberlake

36. "Your Smiling Face" by James Taylor

37. "King Tut" (from *Saturday Night Live*) by Steve Martin

38. "Sunshine on My Shoulders" by John Denver

Photos: In the venue can be photos from my life for family and friends to enjoy. I especially like the ones from our vacations with all seventeen of us. You may want to show the two-hundred-page album of "Grandpa's photos" I gave you at Christmas 2023.

Memory table with significant "physical things" from my life: If you want, you could have a "memory table" and display some of the books I authored, a few of the films I made, my Personal Mission Statement, one of my talks or workshops, one or two of my family journals, a few of my letters, the family history I wrote, my juggling balls, a few of my cartoons, my favorite piano music, my naval cap, my Emmy, my tennis racket, and boxing gloves.

 P.S.: Remember to contact our attorney about our wills: Leah Morabito: Lmorabito@mcmillanmetro.com.

* * * * *

"WE REMEMBER THEM" BY SYLVAN KAMENS & RABBI JACK RIEMER (READING #1)

At the rising sun and at its going down; We remember them.

At the blowing of the wind and in the chill of winter; We remember them.

At the opening of the buds and in the rebirth of spring; We remember them.

At the blueness of the skies and in the warmth of summer; We remember them.

At the rustling of the leaves and in the beauty of the autumn; We remember them.

At the beginning of the year and when it ends; We remember them.

As long as we live, they too will live, for they are now a part of us as We remember them.

When we are weary and in need of strength; We remember them.

When we are lost and sick at heart; We remember them.

When we have decisions that are difficult to make; We remember them.

When we have joy we crave to share; We remember them.

When we have achievements that are based on theirs; We remember them.

For as long as we live, they too will live, for they are now a part of us as, We remember them.

"OUR LIVES MATTER" BY M. MAUREEN KILLORAN (READING #2)

We come together from the diversity of our grieving,

to gather in the warmth of this community

giving stubborn witness to our belief that

in times of sadness, there is room for laughter.

In times of darkness, there always will be light.

May we hold fast to the conviction

that what we do with our lives matters

and that a caring world is possible after all.

"The Wolf Credo" by Del Goetz (Reading #3)

(Gail and I suggest each grandchild read one line aloud.)

Respect the elders
Teach the young
Cooperate with the pack

Play when you can
Hunt when you must
Rest in-between

Share your affections
Voice your feelings
Leave your mark

ACKNOWLEDGMENTS

In the same way a good death is invariably a team effort, this book would never have been possible without countless people helping me in many different ways.

My primary debt is to my family, especially my beloved wife, Gail, to whom the book is dedicated. For nearly a decade, Gail put up with my relentless focus on death and dying as I worked on this book. She read the whole manuscript and gave me helpful feedback. Her guidance, love, and wisdom are nonpareil.

In addition to Gail, I thank my three cherished and accomplished daughters, Kimberly, Christina, and Jennifer, who read the book and gave me useful feedback. The love I receive from my family is ever sustaining. I'm deeply grateful to my three outstanding sons-in-law (Sujay, CJ, and Chase) and my nine adored and adorable grandchildren: Kareena, Neal, JJ, Max, Sammy, Aiden, Connor, Dylan, and Charlie.

Several friends and colleagues went above and beyond to support me, and I am profoundly grateful to them for their generosity. They include (in alphabetical order) Mary Jo Deering, Roger DiSilvestro, Peggy Engel, Adrian Gardner, and my lifelong friend Grant Thompson. They reviewed early drafts of the manuscript and told me that large chunks of it needed to be substantially revised and rewritten, which I then proceeded to do. The honesty of true friends is one of life's many blessings. All are mensches of the highest order. Their constructive and energizing feedback was invaluable.

Many others helped me create this book through their work, conversations, research, writings, and feedback. Among them are (in alphabetical order) Barbara Blaylock, Lowrey Brown, Kim Callinan, Michael

Cordes, Basil Eldadah, Ellen Liu, Beth Morrison, Lee Webster, and David Zinner. I also received help and inspiration from Howard Berg, Ericka Cameron, Glenn Easton, Tracey Gendron, Mardy Grothe, Steve King, Roz Kipping, Morris Klein, Isabel Knight, Hank Levine, Diane MacEachern, Tara Perez, Melanie Raine, and Eleanor Tanno.

My heartfelt gratitude goes to all those who shared their personal stories with me, including Ann Bennet, Debbie Davenport, Peggy Engel, Barry Gorman, Steve King, Roz Kipping, Ellen Liu, Diane MacEachern, Dave Nathan, Patti Steckler, Meredith Taylor, Grant Thompson, and many others who prefer to remain anonymous.

I appreciate the editing skills of Wendy A. Jordan, who did an excellent job editing the whole manuscript.

For their inspiration and support, I thank my amazing friends and colleagues at the Bethesda Metro Area Village (BMAV), Montgomery Hospice and Prince George's Hospice (MHI), the Maryland Office of Cemetery Oversight (MOCO), the Funeral Consumers Alliance of Maryland and Environs (FCAME), the Green Burial Association of Maryland (GBAM), and the Washington Area Villages Exchange (WAVE). I especially want to single out (in alphabetical order) Lynn Barclay, Rachel Bayard, Barbara Blaylock, Jane Boynton, Marlene Bradford, Barbara Brown, Hanne Caraher, Naomi Collins, Bruce Coolidge, Michael Cordes, Mary Jo Deering, Reid Detchon, Dawn Doebler, Jennifer Downs, Mike Franch, Cele Garrett, Barry Gorman, Elizabeth Haile, Robin Hessey, Kim Holcomb, Elyse Jacob, Shady Jadali, Dick Jung, Diana Kitt, Diane Kuwamura, Elma Levy, Ann Mitchell, Cecilia Otero, Jeanne Parker, Frank Porter, Jennifer Plude, Laurie Pross, Debbie Rappazzo, Justin Reaves, David Schrier, Shobhana Sharma, Cornelia Stronge, Stephanie Sutton, Barbara Wiss, and David Zinner.

Over the years, I owe incalculable thanks to fellow authors who have deepened my understanding of death and dying issues. I have benefited enormously from the insights of the following distinguished researchers, doctors, scholars, and activists, each the author of a landmark book on death and dying. They are (in alphabetical order) John Abraham, Marc Agronin, Louise Aronson, Shahid Aziz, Ernest Becker, Shoshana Berger, Amy Bloom, Katy Butler, Ira Byock, Daniel Callahan, Kimberly

Callinan, Lisa Carlson, Barbara Coombs Lee, Joan Didion, Caitlin Doughty, L. S. Dugdale, Hank Dunn, Katie Engelhart, Atul Gawande, Drew Gilpin Faust, Tracey Gendron, Jeff Greenberg, Samuel Harrington, Michael Hebb, Christopher Hitchens, Derek Humphry, Paul Kalanithi, Barbara Karnes, David Kessler, Paul Menzel, BJ Miller, Jessica Mitford, Dan Morhaim, Sarah Murray, Ann Neumann, Sherwin Nuland, Steven Petrow, Thaddeus Pope, Sunita Puri, Tom Pyszczynski, Timothy Quill, Diane Rehm, Gail Rubin, Judith Schwarz, Phyllis Shacter, Lonny Shavelson, Josh Slocum, Sheldon Solomon, Cory Taylor, Sallie Tisdale, Haider Warraich, Irvin Yalom, and Jessica Nutik Zitter. I'm deeply grateful to each of these luminaries and salute them for their inspiration, creativity, and diligence.

I want to acknowledge the writers, thinkers, leaders, and activists who have shaped my life with their wisdom. They have not necessarily written about death and dying, but they have influenced me in vital ways and thus helped shape this book. In particular, I want to thank (in alphabetical order) Joshua Becker, Arthur Brooks, Stephen R. Covey, Mihaly Csikszentmihalyi, Angela Duckworth, Carol Dweck, Viktor Frankl, Maria Garcia, Anu Garg, Adam Grant, Mardy Grothe, Ryan Holiday, Liesl Johnson, Cynthia Meyer, Cal Newport, and Martin Seligman.

Finally, I'm grateful to the team at Rowman & Littlefield, especially Jacquie Flynn, Victoria Shi, and Crystal Branson, for believing in and publishing this book.

* * * * *

All proceeds from this book go to fund scholarships for students at American University, where I taught for fourteen years following my thirty-year career as a wildlife and conservation filmmaker.

Notes

Preface

1. Many researchers believe that the fear of death influences every facet of our lives. For example, see Ernest Becker, *The Denial of Death* (New York: The Free Press, 1973), and Sheldon Solomon, Jeff Greenberg, and Tom Pyszczynski, *On the Role of Death in Life: The Worm at the Core* (New York: Random House, 2015).

Introduction

1. BJ Miller and Shoshana Berger, *A Beginner's Guide to the End: Practical Advice for Living Life and Facing Death* (New York: Simon & Schuster, 2019), 392.

2. Sarah Murray, *Making an Exit: From the Magnificent to the Macabre—How We Dignify the Dead* (New York: St. Martin's Press, 2011), 135.

3. The Aging Well group is part of the Bethesda Metro Area Village (BMAV) in Bethesda, Maryland, where I live. BMAV is, in turn, part of the growing village movment in this country. I founded the Aging Well group in 2017, and we meet monthly to discuss issues relating to aging, death, and dying.

4. The Arnold Toynbee quote comes from Katharine Esty, *Eightysomethings: A Practical Guide to Letting Go, Aging Well, and Finding Unexpected Happiness* (New York: Skyhorse Publishing, 2019), 145.

5. Ira Byock, *The Best Care Possible: A Physician's Quest to Transform Care through the End of Life* (New York: Avery, 2012), 6.

6. Drew Gilpin Faust, *The Republic of Suffering: Death and the American Civil War* (New York: Vintage Books, 2008), 9.

7. The Elisabeth Kübler-Ross quote comes from Michael Hebb, *Let's Talk about Death over Dinner* (Boston, MA: Da Capo Press, Hachette Book Group, 2018), 12.

8. I wrote about this in my memoir *Confessions of a Wildlife Filmmaker* (Philadelphia, PA: Bluefield Publishing, 2015), 97.

9. Ira Byock, *The Best Care Possible: A Physician's Quest to Transform Care through the End of Life* (New York: Avery, 2012), 1.

10. This quote is from Dr. Mardy Grothe's excellent weekly newsletter, *Dr. Mardy's Quotes of the Week*, published May 8, 2022.

11. BJ Miller and Shoshana Berger, *A Beginner's Guide to the End: Practical Advice for Living Life and Facing Death* (New York: Simon & Schuster, 2019), xii.

12. Fortunately, my mother-in-law had a do-not-resuscitate (DNR) order in place, and her final days were with hospice care, not in a hospital.

13. But see https://www.capc.org/blog/palliative-care-and-hospice-education-and -training-act-pcheta-reintroduced-in-the-senate/.

14. See www.thelancet.com.

15. I'm grateful to Dr. Jessica Nutik Zitter for this phrase. See her book *Extreme Measures: Finding a Better Path to the End of Life* (New York: Penguin Random House, 2017).

16. I'm grateful to Katy Butler's book, *The Art of Dying Well: A Practical Guide to a Good End of Life* (New York: Scribner, 2020), for bringing this poll to my attention. Lis Hamel, Bryan Wu, and Mollyann Brodie, "Views and Experiences with End-of-Life Medical Care in the U.S.," Henry J. Kaiser Family Foundation, in partnership with *The Economist*, April 27, 2017, https://www.kff.org/other/report/views-and-experiences-with-end-of -life-medical-care-in-the-u-s/.

CHAPTER 1

1. Drew Gilpin Faust, *This Republic of Suffering: Death and the American Civil War* (New York: Vintage Books, 2008), 10.

2. See https://khn.org/news/home-hospice-care-unexpectedly-burdens-family-care givers/.

3. I'm grateful to Kimberly Callinan, president and CEO of Compassion & Choices, for helping me understand the concept that a good death is the death the dying person wants.

4. I'm grateful to Dr. Sam Harrington for bringing the following study to my attention: Karen Kehl, RN, et al., "Moving toward Peace: An Analysis of the Concept of a Good Death," *American Journal of Hospice and Palliative Care* 23, no. 4 (2006): 277–86. She concluded that the attributes of a good death were (in order of decreasing importance) being in control, being comfortable, having a sense of closure, being valued as a person, trusting one's care providers, recognizing the impending death, honoring beliefs, minimizing the burden, optimizing relationships, utilizing the appropriate amount of technology, leaving a legacy, and being cared for by family. Dr. Harrington points out that these attributes of a good death are usually inconsistent with an institutionalized death associated with aggressive medical treatments.

5. Barbara Coombs Lee, *Finish Strong: Putting Your Priorities First at Life's End* (Portland, OR: Compassion & Choices, 2019), 3.

6. For more on this topic, see my book *Finding Meaning and Success: Living a Fulfilled and Productive Life* (Washington, DC: Rowman & Littlefield, 2021).

7. Barbara Coombs Lee, *Finish Strong: Putting Your Priorities First at Life's End* (Portland, OR: Compassion & Choices, 2019), 5.

8. Atul Gawande, *Being Mortal: Medicine and What Matters in the End* (New York: Henry Holt and Company, 2014), 1–10.

9. Ira Byock, *The Best Care Possible: A Physician's Quest to Transform Care through the End of Life* (New York: Avery, 2012), 10.

10. I'm grateful to Althea Hachuck, a patient advocate and end-of-life–care expert with Final Exit Network for this story. She wrote about it at length in an essay for the website KevinMD.com on April 19, 2022. Her essay was called, "A Bad Death: The Importance of Truth-Telling at End-of-Life."

11. L. S. Dugdale, *The Lost Art of Dying: Reviving Forgotten Wisdom* (New York: Harper Collins, 2020).

12. Brendan Reilly and Arthur Evans, "Much Ado about (Doing) Nothing," *Annals of Internal Medicine* 150, no. 4 (February 17, 2009): 270–71.

13. BJ Miller and Shoshana Berger, *A Beginner's Guide to the End: Practical Advice for Living Life and Facing Death* (New York: Simon & Schuster, 2019), 119.

14. I'm grateful to Barbara Coombs Lee for the section on why doctors overtreat. She describes the problem eloquently in her book *Finish Strong*, and I have used her analysis.

15. Richard B. Stuart, "Organized Medicine Wants to Control Your Death," The Good Death Society Blog, April 24, 2022.

16. Atul Gawande, *Being Mortal: Medicine and What Matters in the End* (New York: Henry Holt and Company, 2014).

17. See www.thebetterend.com.

18. Dan Morhaim, *Preparing for a Better End: Expert Lessons on Death and Dying for You and Your Loved Ones* (Baltimore, MD: Johns Hopkins Press, 2020).

19. Katy Butler, *Knocking on Heaven's Door: The Path to a Better Way of Death* (New York: Scribner, 2013).

20. December 14, 2020, https://blogs.umsl.edu/news/2020/12/14/lila-moersch/.)

21. "The Illness Is Bad Enough. The Hospital May Be Even Worse," *New York Times*, August 3, 2018.

22. "Some Hospitals Producing 'epidemic of immobility,'" *The Washington Post*, October 15, 2019.

23. Dr. Samuel Harrington, *At Peace: Choosing a Good Death after a Long Life* (New York and Boston: Hachette Book Group, 2018).

24. LS Dugdale, *The Lost Art of Dying: Reviving Forgotten Wisdom* (New York: Harper Collins, 2020).

25. For example, see Martin Makary, and others, "Frailty as a Predictor of Surgical Outcomes in Older Patients," *Journal of the American College of Surgeons* 210, no. 6 (2010): 901–8.

26. Hank Dunn, *Hard Choices for Loving People: CPR, Feeding Tubes, Palliative Care, Comfort Measures, and the Patient with a Serious Illness* (Naples, FL: Quality of Life Publishing Co., 2016), 7, www.hankdunn.com.

27. Hank Dunn, *Hard Choices for Loving People: CPR, Feeding Tubes, Palliative Care, Comfort Measures, and the Patient with a Serious Illness* (Naples, FL: Quality of Life Publishing Co., 2016), 8, www.hankdunn.com.

28. Hank Dunn, *Hard Choices for Loving People: CPR, Feeding Tubes, Palliative Care, Comfort Measures, and the Patient with a Serious Illness* (Naples, FL: Quality of Life Publishing Co., 2016), 56, www.hankdunn.com.

29. Barbara Coombs Lee, *Finish Strong: Putting Your Priorities First at Life's End* (Portland, OR: Compassion & Choices, 2019), 13.

30. L. S. Dugdale, *The Lost Art of Dying: Reviving Forgotten Wisdom* (New York: Harper Collins, 2020), 196.

31. Dan Morhaim, *Preparing for a Better End: Expert Lessons on Death and Dying for You and Your Loved Ones* (Baltimore, MD: Johns Hopkins Press, 2020), 51.

32. Dan Morhaim, *Preparing for a Better End: Expert Lessons on Death and Dying for You and Your Loved Ones* (Baltimore, MD: Johns Hopkins Press, 2020), 37.

33. Dr. Samuel Harrington, *At Peace: Choosing a Good Death after a Long Life* (New York and Boston: Hachette Book Group, 2018), 7.

34. Barbara Coombs Lee, *Finish Strong: Putting Your Priorities First at Life's End* (Portland, OR: Compassion & Choices, 2019), 127.

35. Peter Tyson, "The Hippocratic Oath Today: Hippocratic Oath: Modern Version," March 21, 2001, pbs.org/wgbh/nova/body/hippocratic-oath-today.html.

36. Jessica Nutik Zitter, *Extreme Measures: Finding a Better Path to the End of Life* (New York: Penguin Random House, 2017), 33.

37. Jessica Nutik Zitter, *Extreme Measures: Finding a Better Path to the End of Life* (New York: Penguin Random House, 2017), 49.

38. Adam Singer, Daniella Meeker, Joan Teno, et al., "Symptom Trends in the Last Year of Life from 1998 to 2010: A Cohort Study," *Annals of Internal Medicine* 162, no. 3 (2015): 175–83.

39. Jessica Nutik Zitter, *Extreme Measures: Finding a Better Path to the End of Life* (New York: Penguin Random House, 2017), 200.

40. Irvin Yalom, *Staring at the Sun: Overcoming the Dread of Death* (London: Piatkus, 2008), 120.

41. Barbara Karnes, RN, *The Final Act of Living: Reflections of a Long-Time Hospice Nurse* (Vancouver, WA: Barbara Karnes Books, 2012).

42. Ken Murray, "How Doctors Die: It's Not Like the Rest of Us, but It Should Be," *Zocolo Public Square*, November 30, 2011.

43. Vyjeyanthi Periyakoil, Eric Neri, Ann Fong, and Helena Kraemer, "Do Unto Others: Doctor's Personal End-of-Life Resuscitation Preferences and Their Attitudes toward Advance Directives," *PLOS ONE* 9, no. 5 (2014): e98246.

44. Saul Becker, Norman Johnson, Sean Altekruse, and Leora Horwitz, "Association of Occupation as a Physician with Likelihood of Dying in a Hospital," *Journal of the American Medical Association* 315, no. 3 (2016): 301–3.

45. Jessica Nutik Zitter, *Extreme Measures: Finding a Better Path to the End of Life* (New York: Penguin Random House, 2017), 206.

46. Sunita Puri, *That Good Night: Life and Medicine in the Eleventh Hour* (New York: Viking, 2019), 260.

47. Dan Morhaim, *Preparing for a Better End: Expert Lessons on Death and Dying for You and Your Loved Ones* (Baltimore, MD: Johns Hopkins Press, 2020), 80.

48. Haider Warraich, *Modern Death: How Medicine Changed the End of Life* (New York: St. Martin's Press, 2017), 278.

49. Ann Neumann, *The Good Death: An Exploration of Dying America* (Boston, MA: Beacon Press, 2016), 44.

50. BJ Miller and Shoshana Berger, *A Beginner's Guide to the End: Practical Advice for Living Life and Facing Death* (New York: Simon & Schuster, 2019), 268.

51. Jessica Nutik Zitter, *Extreme Measures: Finding a Better Path to the End of Life* (New York: Penguin Random House, 2017), 270.

52. Barbara Coombs Lee, *Finish Strong: Putting Your Priorities First at Life's End* (Portland, OR: Compassion & Choices, 2019), 63.

53. Jessica Nutik Zitter, *Extreme Measures: Finding a Better Path to the End of Life* (New York: Penguin Random House, 2017), 86.

54. Jessica Nutik Zitter, *Extreme Measures: Finding a Better Path to the End of Life* (New York: Penguin Random House, 2017), 86.

55. Victoria Sweet, *Slow Medicine: The Way to Healing* (New York: Riverhead Books, 2017).

56. Katy Butler, *The Art of Dying Well: A Practical Guide to a Good End of Life* (New York: Scribner, 2019), 6.

57. Jessica Nutik Zitter, *Extreme Measures: Finding a Better Path to the End of Life* (New York: Penguin Random House, 2017), 145.

58. Frank Bruni, *The Beauty of Dusk: On Vision Lost and Found* (New York: Simon & Schuster, 2022).

59. Sunita Puri, *That Good Night: Life and Medicine in the Eleventh Hour* (New York: Viking, 2019), 291.

CHAPTER 2

1. Sallie Tisdale, *Advice for Future Corpses: A Practical Perspective on Death and Dying* (New York: Touchstone, 2018), 14.

2. L. S. Dugdale, *The Lost Art of Dying: Reviving Forgotten Wisdom* (New York: Harper Collins, 2020).

3. Private email from Dr. Barry Gorman to the author on November 14, 2021.

4. For more on this topic, see my book *Finding Meaning and Success: Living a Fulfilled and Productive Life* (Washington, DC: Rowman & Littlefield, 2021).

5. Katy Butler, *The Art of Dying Well: A Practical Guide to a Good End of Life* (New York: Scribner, 2019), 6.

6. Louise Aronson, *Elderhood: Redefining Aging, Transforming Medicine, Reimagining Life* (London: Bloomsbury Publishing, 2019).

7. See https://www.theatlantic.com/ideas/archive/2023/01/harvard-happiness-study -relationships/672753/.

8. See https://www.ncbi.nlm.nih.gov/pmc/articles/PMC7529452/.

9. See https://newsnetwork.mayoclinic.org/discussion/poor-diet-and-lack-of-exercise -accelerate-the-onset-of-age-related-conditions-in-mice/.

10. See https://www.cancer.org/about-us/what-we-do/encouraging-prevention.html.

11. Old-old age, when we are frail, brings challenges, but this is not the same as saying that being old is always a problem. Age alone is a poor indicator of health because young-old age, starting at about 60 or 65, can go on for many years if we take good care of ourselves. One key point to remember in this discussion (and I am grateful to Dr. Tracey Gendron at the Virginia Center on Aging for bringing this to my attention) is the impact

of social determinants of health, like living in poverty and having access to health care (which is a privilege and unattainable for some). We must also be careful that describing the desire to delay the loss of autonomy, indignities, etc., not be viewed as "ableist." We must never discriminate against or devalue people with disabilities. Many people of all ages live their whole lives without autonomy and in states of physical pain. However, that doesn't mean that they don't have quality of life or that they don't value life. Also, it is good to remind ourselves that while getting older doesn't necessarily mean deterioration, a lowering of our quality of life should be expected at some point because we are all mortal. Aging itself doesn't equate to deterioration since it involves growth as well as decline, but not acknowledging our mortality in relation to aging produces fear of death. I discuss this more in the next section, "Growth at the End of Life."

12. See https://en.wikipedia.org/wiki/Erikson%27s_stages_of_psychosocial _development#Ninth_stage.

13. Guiseppe Passarino, Francesco De Rango, and Albert Montesanto, "Human Longevity: Genetics or Lifestyle? It Takes Two to Tango," *Immunity & Ageing* 13, no. 1 (2016): 1–6.

14. For more on this topic, see the book by Tracey Gendron, PhD, *Ageism Unmasked: Exploring Age Bias and How to End It* (Lebanon, NH: Steerforth Press, 2022).

15. See my book *Finding Meaning and Success; Living a Fulfilled and Productive Life* (Washington, DC: Rowman & Littlefield, 2021).

16. https://www.nytimes.com/2015/04/12/opinion/sunday/david-brooks-the-moral -bucket-list.html.

17. Psychologist Martin Seligman has written extensively on this topic. For example, see his book *Flourish: A Visionary New Understanding of Happiness and Well-being.*

18. I write about finding meaning and purpose extensively in my book *Finding Meaning and Success; Living a Fulfilled and Productive Life* (Washington, DC: Rowman & Littlefield, 2021).

19. If you want to see my personal mission statement, send me an email (christopher.n.palmer@gmail.com), and I will send it to you.

20. Lydia Dugdale, "The Lost Art of Dying Well," *Columbia Magazine* Winter 2020–2021, 36.

21. https://time.com/4475628/the-new-science-of-exercise/.

22. See Marc Agronin, *The End of Old Age: Living a Longer, More Purposeful Life* (Boston, MA: De Capo Press, 2018).

23. On the topic of living with purpose, I recommend reading pages 125–28 in Atul Gwande's 2014 book *Being Mortal: Medicine and What Matters in the End.*

24. Dr. Louise Aronson, *Elderhood: Redefining Aging, Transforming Medicine, Reimagining Life* (London: Bloomsbury Publishing, 2019), 9.

25. Dr. Becca Levy, *Breaking the Age Code: How Your Beliefs about Aging Determine How Well & Long You Live* (New York: Harper Collins, 2022).

26. Becca R. Levy, Martin D. Slade, Suzanne R. Kunkel, and Stanislav V. Kasl, "Longevity Increased by Positive Self-Perception of Aging," *Journal of Personality and Social Psychology* 83, no. 2 (2002): 261.

27. See also Paula Span, "How Ageism Can Take Years Off Seniors' Lives," *New York Times*, April 26, 2022.

28. A valuable book on the topic of aging well is by Richard Siegel and Rabbi Laura Geller, entitled *Getting Good at Getting Older* (Millburn, NJ: Behrman House, 2017).

29. See https://www.nih.gov/about-nih/what-we-do/nih-almanac/national-institute -aging-nia.

30. Robert N. Butler, "Psychiatry and the Elderly: An Overview," *The American Journal of Psychiatry* 132, no. 9 (1975): 894.

31. Tracey Gendron, PhD, *Ageism Unmasked: Exploring Age Bias and How to End It* (Lebanon, NH: Steerforth Press, 2022), 8.

32. Ashton Applewhite, *This Chair Rocks: A Manifesto against Ageism* (New York: Celadon Books, 2016), 98.

33. Tracey Gendron, PhD, *Ageism Unmasked: Exploring Age Bias and How to End It* (Lebanon, NH: Steerforth Press, 2022), 11.

34. James Hillman, *The Force of Character and the Lasting Life* (New York: Random House, 1999).

35. An excellent book exploring this area more is Mindy Greenstein and Jimmie Holland's book *Lighter as We Go: Virtues, Character Strengths, and Aging* (Oxford, UK: Oxford University Press, 2015).

36. Tracey Gendron, PhD, *Ageism Unmasked: Exploring Age Bias and How to End It* (Lebanon, NH: Steerforth Press, 2022), 5.

37. Dr. Robert Butler, *Why Survive? Being Old in America* (Baltimore, MD: Johns Hopkins University Press, 1975), 76.

38. Marc Agronin, MD, *The End of Old Age: Living a Longer, More Purposeful Life* (Boston, MA: De Capo Press, 2018), 135–38.

39. Marc Agronin, MD, *The End of Old Age: Living a Longer, More Purposeful Life* (Boston, MA: De Capo Press, 2018).

40. https://www.orderofthegooddeath.com/death-positive-movement/.

41. Cory Taylor, *Dying: A Memoir* (New York: W. W. Norton & Company, 2017), 12.

42. See www.deathcafe.com.

43. https://deathoverdinner.org/.

44. See Michael Hebb, *Let's Talk about Death (over Dinner): An Invitation and Guide to Life's Most Important Conversation* (Boston, MA: Da Capo Press, 2018).

CHAPTER 3

1. Steven Petrow, *Stupid Things I Won't Do When I Get Old: A Highly Judgmental, Unapologetically Honest Accounting of All the Things Our Elders Are Doing Wrong* (New York: Citadel Press, 2021), 125.

2. Private email to author from Dave Nathan on July 1, 2023.

3. I highly recommend Maria Gracia's daily e-newsletter. Go to GetOrganizedNow.com.

4. See https://www.becomingminimalist.com/.

5. Joshua Becker, *The Minimalist Home: A Room-by-Room Guide to a Decluttered, Refocused Life* (Colorado Springs, CO: Waterbrook, 2018), 7.

6. Katy Butler, in her book *The Art of Dying Well*, calls simplification "a survival skill" (page 41).

7. See https://www.legalzoom.com/articles/estate-planning-statistics.

8. BJ Miller and Shoshana Berger, *A Beginner's Guide to the End: Practical Advice for Living Life and Facing Death* (New York: Simon & Schuster, 2019), 51.

9. Your lawyer may also advise on alternatives to a legal will, such as a trust or transfer of death designations.

10. https://www.washingtonpost.com/wellness/2022/11/20/death-red-tape-bureaucracy-finances/.

CHAPTER 4

1. Private email dated September 17, 2022, to author.

2. Dr. Dan Morhaim, "Why Your Patients Need Advance Care Plans," *Medical Economics*, July 14, 2022. https://www.medicaleconomics.com/view/why-your-patients-need-advance-care-plans.

3. Dan Morhaim, *Preparing for a Better End: Expert Lessons on Death and Dying for You and Your Loved Ones* (Baltimore, MD: Johns Hopkins Press, 2020).

4. See https://www.nia.nih.gov/health/frequently-asked-questions-about-palliative-care?utm_source=nia-eblast&utm_medium=email&utm_campaign=caregiving-20220324.

5. See Dan Morhaim, MD, "We Need to Talk About Death in 2022," Smerconish.com in 2022.

6. See Dan Morhaim, MD, "Why Your Patients Need Advance Care Plans," *Medical Economics*, July 14, 2022.

7. I recommend the Stanford letter as another approach to preparation and planning on end-of-life issues: med.stanford.edu/letter.html.

8. Dr. Shahid Aziz, *Courageous Conversations on Dying: The Gift of Palliative Care* (2018), 78.

9. For more on Dr. Eleanor Tanno, see https://advancedirectivemd.com/about/.

10. Dan Morhaim, MD, is an emergency-medicine physician, a former Maryland state legislator (1995–2019), and a health-care consultant, and his 2020 book is *Preparing for a Better End* (Baltimore, MD: Johns Hopkins University Press, 2020), www.thebetterend.com.

11. Dan Morhaim, MD, "We Need to Talk about Death in 2022," Smerconish.com.

12. I wrote that people "suffer" with dementia, and I used the phrase "patients with dementia." I also wrote that a person with dementia faces the terrifying prospect of becoming a dysfunctional and different person. However, there is a fairly strong movement to reframe this language and talk instead about people "living" with dementia and not referring to them as perpetual "patients" in order to destigmatize the experience. This is important because it also contributes to ableism and makes an assumption that having dementia means life is not worth living, which may not be accurate for all people.

13. See alz.org.

14. B. Z. Aminoff and A. Adunsky, "Dying Dementia Patients: Too Much Suffering, Too Little Palliation," *American Journal of Hospital Palliative Care* 22, no. 5 (September–October 2005): 344–48.

15. https://www.compassionandchoices.org/docs/default-source/default-document-library/dementia-provision-only-final-6-29-20-pdf.pdf?sfvrsn=2aebdcb5_2&utm_campaign=natwebinar&utm_source=communityengagement&sourceid=1079767&utm_medium=email&UTM_content=AEN5-follow-up&emci=37c6a37c-c03a-ee11-a3f1-00224832eb73&emdi=818c8280-fa3a-ee11-a3f1-00224832eb73&ceid=1198209.

16. So many people are getting Alzheimer's and other dementia that it is vital to add a dementia provision to your advance directive. The best one I've seen comes from Compassion & Choices: https://values-tool.compassionandchoices.org/?_ga=2.50574441.1939191242.1650747017-1614916080.1634565379). I urge you to answer the questions online and get some peace of mind by doing so.

17. I am grateful to the listserv of the American Clinicians Academy on Medical Aid in Dying for the legal information from attorney Kathryn Tucker.

18. Althea Halchuck, Final Exit Network consultant, "'Wrongful Life' Lawsuits," Final Exit Network newsletter (Summer 2022).

19. See https://en.wikipedia.org/wiki/Patient_Self-Determination_Act.

20. See Faye Girsh, "Interview with Faye Girsh—An Activist for the Right to a Peaceful Death," interview by Scott Douglas Jacobsen, The Good Death Society Blog, June 12, 2022.

21. Jim Parker, "Health Care Orgs Face Liability If End-of-Life Wishes Not Upheld," June 17, 2022, HospiceNews.com, https://hospicenews.com/2022/06/17/health-care-orgs-face-liability-if-end-of-life-wishes-not-upheld/.

22. For example, see Dr. Daniela Lamas, "When Faced with Death, People Often Change Their Minds," *New York Times*, January 3, 2022.

23. Jessica Nutik Zitter, *Extreme Measures: Finding a Better Path to the End of Life* (New York: Penguin Random House, 2017), 134.

24. Barbara Coombs Lee, *Finish Strong: Putting Your Priorities First at Life's End* (Portland, OR: Compassion & Choices, 2019), 26, 27, 60.

25. Dr. Atul Gawande, *Being Mortal: Medicine and What Matters in the End* (New York: Henry Holt and Company, Metropolitan Books, 2014), 177.

26. Dr. Shahid Aziz, *Courageous Conversations on Dying: the Gift of Palliative Care* (2018), 11, 20.

27. See Dan Morhaim, MD, "Filling Out Free Forms Can Fix Medicare," April 1, 2023, https://www.smerconish.com/exclusive-content/filling-out-free-forms-can-fix-medicare/.

28. Dr. Shahid Aziz stated this in a workshop that I attended in August 2022, while obtaining a certificate in end-of-life care with Montgomery Hospice and Prince George's Hospice in Maryland.

29. See The Report of the Lancet Commission on the Value of Death: Bringing Death Back into Life, published January 31, 2022, on www.thelancet.com.

30. See Jessica Nutik Zitter, *Extreme Measures: Finding a Better Path to the End of Life* (New York: Penguin Random House, 2017), 143.

31. Dr. Atul Gawande, *Being Mortal: Medicine and What Matters in the End* (New York: Henry Holt and Company, Metropolitan Books, 2014), 178.

32. Sunita Puri, *That Good Night: Life and Medicine in the Eleventh Hour* (New York: Viking, 2019), 267.

33. See https://theconversationproject.org.

34. Jessica Nutik Zitter, *Extreme Measures: Finding a Better Path to the End of Life* (New York: Penguin Random House, 2017), 107.

35. BJ Miller and Shoshana Berger, *A Beginner's Guide to the End: Practical Advice for Living Life and Facing Death* (New York: Simon & Schuster, 2019), 108.

36. Dr. Samuel Harrington, *At Peace: Choosing a Good Death after a Long Life* (New York and Boston: Hachette Book Group, 2018), 151.

37. BJ Miller and Shoshana Berger, *A Beginner's Guide to the End: Practical Advice for Living Life and Facing Death* (New York: Simon & Schuster, 2019), 92.

38. Dr. Atul Gawande, *Being Mortal: Medicine and What Matters in the End* (New York: Henry Holt and Company, Metropolitan Books, 2014), 1.

39. Dr. Louise Aronson, *Elderhood: Redefining Aging, Transforming Medicine, Reimagining Life* (London: Bloomsbury Publishing, 2019), 300.

40. Ira Byock, *The Best Care Possible: A Physician's Quest to Transform Care through the End of Life* (New York: Avery, 2012).

41. Jessica Nutik Zitter, *Extreme Measures: Finding a Better Path to the End of Life* (New York: Penguin Random House, 2017), 295.

42. Rosalind Kipping, personal email to the author, July 29, 2021.

43. You may have heard of the saying, "Don't take your organs to Heaven. They are needed here on Earth." There is much truth to it. Organ donation is a wonderful way to continue a living legacy. I recommend that people designate themselves as organ donors. Organ transplants have saved and improved thousands of lives, but there continues to be a shortage of donors. Medical advances allow a wide variety of donations, from cornea and skin tissues to hearts, lungs, livers, and kidneys. Even those who die at an advanced age or with an underlying health condition can be donors. While I believe that you should designate all organs for donation, a skilled advisor will help to determine what is appropriate in each individual case. For information on the details of the organ donation process, see organdonor.gov and Donate Life America (donatelife.net). Another possibility is whole body donation to medical science. This is usually arranged through a medical school and needs to be arranged for in advance. There's no cost for this, and it helps medical education and research.

44. BJ Miller and Shoshana Berger, *A Beginner's Guide to the End: Practical Advice for Living Life and Facing Death* (New York: Simon & Schuster, 2019), 43.

45. Dr. Samuel Harrington, *At Peace: Choosing a Good Death after a Long Life* (New York and Boston: Hachette Book Group, 2018), 109.

46. Dr. Samuel Harrington, *At Peace: Choosing a Good Death after a Long Life* (New York and Boston: Hachette Book Group, 2018), 118.

47. Dr. Samuel Harrington, *At Peace: Choosing a Good Death after a Long Life* (New York and Boston: Hachette Book Group, 2018), 108.

48. Dr. Samuel Harrington, *At Peace: Choosing a Good Death after a Long Life* (New York and Boston: Hachette Book Group, 2018), 115.

CHAPTER 5

1. I write more about "rippling" in the Epilogue.

2. See https://www.joincake.com/blog/legacy-quotes/.

3. See https://aucklandunitarian.org.nz/podcast/20191110_RevClayNelson_IAm WhatSurvivesMe.pdf.

4. I'm grateful to author, speaker, and humorist Ron Culberson for inspiring me with this idea. He is the author of the book *Do it Well. Make it Fun* (Austin, TX: Greenleaf Book Group Press, 2012).

5. Rabbi Steve Leder, *For You When I'm Gone: Twelve Essential Questions to Tell a Life Story* (New York: Avery, 2022).

6. Poem by Mary Oliver called "The Summer Day."

7. I have written three memoirs (*Shooting in the Wild, Confessions of a Wildlife Filmmaker,* and *Open Heart*) and owe a debt of gratitude to the following authors and books for their guidance and wisdom: *Your Legacy in a Book* by Caroline Lambert, *For All Time* by Charley Kempthorne, *Writing Family Histories and Memoirs* by Kirk Polking, *Your Life as Story* by Tristine Rainer, and *Fast-Draft Your Memoir* by Rachel Herron. My advice on how to write a memoir largely comes from these authors, as well as from my own experience.

CHAPTER 6

1. See https://medlineplus.gov/caregiverhealth.html?utm_source=newsletter&utm _campaign=sep15.

2. See https://www.aarp.org/caregiving/basics/info-2020/unpaid-family-caregivers -report.html.

3. See https://www.aplaceformom.com/caregiver-resources/articles/caregiver-statistics.

4. AARP.org/Bulletin, May 2022, page 33.

5. While I talk about becoming "a burden on others," I'm grateful to Dr. Tracey Gendron, author of the excellent book *Ageism Unmasked,* for pointing out to me that the burden narrative can lead to ageism and ableism by fueling fear of dependence and the myth of independence. A healthy balance is interdependence and acknowledging that we always need others to care for us in various ways.

6. AARP.org/Bulletin, May 2022, page 33.

7. Dr. Louise Aronson, *Elderhood: Redefining Aging, Transforming Medicine, Reimagining Life* (London: Bloomsbury Publishing, 2019), 304.

8. Tracey Gendron, *Ageism Unmasked: Exploring Age Bias and How to End It* (Hanover, NH: Steerforth Press, 2022), 137.

9. Janet Bodnar, "Start the Elder Care Conversation," *Kiplinger's Personal Finance,* May 2022.

10. Haider Warraich, *Modern Death: How Medicine Changed the End of Life* (New York: St. Martin's Press, 2017), 178.

11. See https://www.womenshealth.gov/a-z-topics/caregiver-stress.

12. Haider Warraich, *Modern Death: How Medicine Changed the End of Life* (New York: St. Martin's Press, 2017), 209–10.

13. Christopher Hitchens, *Mortality* (New York: Hatchette Book Group, 2012).

14. Steven Petrow, "Cancer Etiquette: It's Long Overdue," *The Washington Post*, June 14, 2022.

CHAPTER 7

1. If you're looking for palliative care in your area, visit the National Hospice and Palliative Care Organization website: https://www.nhpco.org/.

2. Jessica Nutik Zitter, *Extreme Measures: Finding a Better Path to the End of Life* (New York: Penguin Random House, 2017), 299.

3. See https://www.nia.nih.gov/health/frequently-asked-questions-about-palliative-care?utm_source=nia-eblast&utm_medium=email&utm_campaign=caregiving-20220324.

4. See https://www.nhpco.org/.

5. BJ Miller and Shoshana Berger, *A Beginner's Guide to the End: Practical Advice for Living Life and Facing Death* (New York: Simon & Schuster, 2019), 195.

6. Sunita Puri, *That Good Night: Life and Medicine in the Eleventh Hour* (New York: Viking, 2019), 206.

7. Quoted by Dr. Lonny Shavelson in his booklet *Medical Aid in Dying: A Guide for Patients and their Supporters*, published by the American Clinicians Academy on Medical Aid in Dying, 2022, page 21.

8. See https://www.nia.nih.gov/health/frequently-asked-questions-about-palliative-care?utm_source=nia-eblast&utm_medium=email&utm_campaign=caregiving-20220324.

9. An example of an inpatient hospice is Casey House, run by the nonprofit Montgomery Hospice and Prince George's Hospice in Maryland. Casey House has the feel, warmth, and caring of a home. The nursing staff is present 24/7, and doctors are available on call. Full disclosure: I serve on the Board of Montgomery Hospice and Prince George's Hospice.

10. Dr. Samuel Harrington, *At Peace: Choosing a Good Death after a Long Life* (New York and Boston: Hachette Book Group, 2018), 177.

11. Dr. Atul Gawande, *Being Mortal: Medicine and What Matters in the End* (New York: Henry Holt and Company, Metropolitan Books, 2014), 9.

12. Haider Warraich, *Modern Death: How Medicine Changed the End of Life* (New York: St. Martin's Press, 2017), 264.

13. Haider Warraich, *Modern Death: How Medicine Changed the End of Life* (New York: St. Martin's Press, 2017), 264.

14. Jessica Nutik Zitter, *Extreme Measures: Finding a Better Path to the End of Life* (New York: Penguin Random House, 2017), 48.

15. Dr. Samuel Harrington, *At Peace: Choosing a Good Death after a Long Life* (New York and Boston: Hachette Book Group, 2018), 188.

16. Dr. Atul Gawande, *Being Mortal: Medicine and What Matters in the End* (New York: Henry Holt and Company, Metropolitan Books, 2014), 178.

17. Barbara Coombs Lee, *Finish Strong: Putting Your Priorities First at Life's End* (Portland, OR: Compassion & Choices, 2019), 94.

18. Dr. Atul Gawande, *Being Mortal: Medicine and What Matters in the End* (New York: Henry Holt and Company, Metropolitan Books, 2014), 177–78.

19. Closely related to overmedicalization is the concept of iatrongenesis. See https://en.wikipedia.org/wiki/Iatrogenesis. Iatrogenic errors and mistakes by doctors in hospitals are a significant problem.

20. BJ Miller and Shoshana Berger, *A Beginner's Guide to the End: Practical Advice for Living Life and Facing Death* (New York: Simon & Schuster, 2019), 204.

21. Dan Morhaim, *Preparing for a Better End: Expert Lessons on Death and Dying for You and Your Loved Ones* (Baltimore, MD: Johns Hopkins University Press, 2020), 75.

22. Dr. Samuel Harrington, *At Peace: Choosing a Good Death after a Long Life* (New York and Boston: Hachette Book Group, 2018), 192.

23. See Dave Kovaleski's report on August 10, 2021, in FinancialRegulationNews.com.

24. These statistics come from hospice consultant and expert Sue Lyn Schramm. Her website is https://schrammconsulting.com/.

25. Private email to author from Margaret Engel dated October 3, 2023.

26. Haider Warraich, "Most People Now Die at Home. Care Can Be Complex." *The Washington Post*, February 18, 2020.

27. Sunita Puri, *That Good Night: Life and Medicine in the Eleventh Hour* (New York: Viking, 2019).

28. Sunita Puri, *That Good Night: Life and Medicine in the Eleventh Hour* (New York: Viking, 2019), 210.

29. On page 167 of Katy Butler's outstanding 2019 book *The Art of Dying Well*, she writes, "Uncontrolled pain is a common barrier to a peaceful death, currently affecting 61 percent of people in their last year of life."

30. See https://journalofethics.ama-assn.org/article/ama-code-medical-ethics-opinions-care-end-life/2013-12.

31. Melissa Wachterman, Elizabeth Luth, Robert Semco, and Joel Weissman, "Where Americans Die—Is There Really 'No Place Like Home'?," *The New England Journal of Medicine*, March 17, 2022 (and published on March 12, 2022, at NEJM.org).

32. For an overview of death doulas, see Dr. Christina Palmer's GoodRx essay: https://www.goodrx.com/healthcare-access/patient-advocacy/death-doula.

CHAPTER 8

1. See https://www.thegooddeathsocietyblog.net/2021/10/24/what-ways-can-you-die-when-youve-had-enough-of-life/.

2. John Abraham, *How to Get the Death You Want: A Practical and Moral Guide* (Hinesburg, VT: Upper Access Books, 2017), 15.

3. Craig Sechler, filmmaker and a friend of the author's, personal email to the author, November 17, 2011.

4. Timothy Quil, Paul Menzel, Thaddeus Pope, and Judith Schwarz, *Voluntarily Stopping Eating and Drinking: A Compassionate, Widely Available Option for Hastening Death* (Oxford, UK: Oxford University Press, 2021).

5. Timothy Quil, Paul Menzel, Thaddeus Pope, and Judith Schwarz, *Voluntarily Stopping Eating and Drinking: A Compassionate, Widely Available Option for Hastening Death* (Oxford, UK: Oxford University Press, 2021), 129.

6. Samuel Harrington, *At Peace: Choosing a Good Death after a Long Life* (New York and Boston: Hachette Book Group, 2018), 201

7. Samuel Harrington, *At Peace: Choosing a Good Death after a Long Life* (New York and Boston: Hachette Book Group, 2018), 201.

8. Timothy Quil, Paul Menzel, Thaddeus Pope, and Judith Schwarz, *Voluntarily Stopping Eating and Drinking: A Compassionate, Widely Available Option for Hastening Death* (Oxford, UK: Oxford University Press, 2021).

9. Hank Dunn, *Hard Choices for Loving People: CPR, Feeding Tubes, Palliative Care, Comfort Measures, and the Patient with a Serious Illness* (Naples, FL: Quality of Life Publishing, 2016), 58.

10. Phyllis Shacter, *Choosing to Die, a Personal Story: Elective Death by Voluntarily Stopping Eating and Drinking (VSED) in the Face of Degenerative Disease* (self-published, 2017).

11. Phyllis Shacter, *Choosing to Die, a Personal Story: Elective Death by Voluntarily Stopping Eating and Drinking (VSED) in the Face of Degenerative Disease* (self-published, 2017), 15.

12. Phyllis Shacter, *Choosing to Die, a Personal Story: Elective Death by Voluntarily Stopping Eating and Drinking (VSED) in the Face of Degenerative Disease* (self-published, 2017), 77.

13. Timothy Quil, Paul Menzel, Thaddeus Pope, and Judith Schwarz, *Voluntarily Stopping Eating and Drinking: A Compassionate, Widely Available Option for Hastening Death* (Oxford, UK: Oxford University Press, 2021).

14. Diane Rehm, *When My Time Comes: Conversations about Whether Those Who Are Dying Should Have the Right to Determine When Life Should End* (New York: Alfred A. Knopf, 2020).

15. https://compassionandchoices.org/legal-advocacy/past-cases/washington-v-glucksberg-vacco-v-quill.

16. Dr. Aziz, private email correspondence with the author, September 8, 2022.

17. Haider Warraich, *Modern Death: How Medicine Changed the End of Life* (New York: St. Martin's Press, 2017), 254.

18. One of the best guides to medical aid in dying (MAID) is a booklet written in 2022 by Dr. Lonny Shavelson who founded and chairs the American Clinicians Academy on Medical Aid in Dying (ACAMAID). The booklet is entitled, *Medical Aid in Dying: A Guide for Patients and Their Supporters*. See www.ACAMAID.org. ACAMAID is focused on innovating and advancing clinical knowledge and best practices relating to MAID.

19. I'm grateful to Dr. Lonny Shavelson, chair and founder of the American Clinicians Academy on Medical Aid in Dying (ACAMAID), for this definition of medical aid in dying.

20. Percutaneous endoscopic gastrostomy (or PEG for short) is where a tube in inserted surgically through the skin into the stomach wall. Liquid nutritional supplements, water, and medications can be poured into the tube or pumped in by way of a mechanical device.

21. The nonprofit organization Compassion & Choices fights to give people more choices at the end of life and is a strong proponent of medical aid in dying. Kimberly Callinan, the president and CEO of Compassion & Choices, points out accurately that the data I am citing at the top of page 128 comes from what *doctors* report is the reason people choose MAID. In Callinan's experience, however, from talking with patients who want MAID, physical pain *is* a major issue. Studies on breakthrough pain confirm this. The vast majority of individuals who use medical aid in dying are also receiving hospice and palliative care, but they still want the option of medical aid in dyingfor a variety of reasons. In other words, good hospice services and palliative care do not eliminate the need for medical aid in dying as an end-of-life care option. As I have pointed out earlier in the book, breakthrough pain—severe pain that occurs even when a patient is already medicated—remains a nightmare experience for too many. In the National Breakthrough Pain Study, among respondents who had cancer (at all stages), 83.3% reported breakthrough pain. For those cancer patients who experienced breakthrough pain, only 24.1% reported that using some form of pain management worked every time. What Callinan hears directly from terminally ill individuals is that people decide to use MAID for multiple reasons all at once: pain and other symptoms such as breathlessness and nausea, loss of autonomy, and loss of dignity. It is not one reason but rather the totality of what happens to one's body at the end of life. For some people, the side effects of treatments such as chemotherapy or pain medication (sedation, relentless nausea, crushing fatigue, obstructed bowels, to name a few) are just as bad as the agonizing symptoms of the disease. Others want the option of medical aid in dying because they want to try that one last, long-shot treatment with the peace of mind of knowing that if it results in unbearable suffering, they have the option to die peacefully. Only the dying person can determine how much pain and suffering is too much. MAID puts the decision in the hands of the dying person, in consultation with their doctor and loved ones, as it should be for such deeply personal health-care decisions.

22. Kimberly Callinan, president and CEO of Compassion & Choices, accurately points out that while having an experienced doctor or nurse be with the patient may be preferable and helpful for *some* patients, that is not necessary or possible for many who live in rural areas or have doctors or nurses who won't travel. Furthermore, many of the families who choose medical aid in dying do so because they want a private and intimate experience that is not overly medicalized. Patients should be given the risks and options and be allowed to decide what is in their best interest. Many patients use the option of medical aid in dying successfully without a doctor or nurse present. Again, it should be the patient's choice.

23. See https://notdeadyet.org/.

24. As a counterweight to Not Dead Yet, see US for Autonomy: https://www.unforautonomy.org.

25. This information comes from David C. Leven, executive director of End of Life Choices New York.

26. I'm grateful to Kim Callinan, president and CEO of Compassion & Choices, for this information on people having to self-pay (or not) for medical aid in dying.

27. See https://ohiooptions.org/brittany-maynards-story-and-testimony/.

28. The following Swiss organizations can also give you information on their criteria and what is needed: Dignitas: www.dignitas.ch/index.php?lang=en; Pegasos: www.pegasos-association.com; Lifecircle + the Eternal SPIRIT Foundation: https://www.lifecircle.ch/en/.

29. See https://www.exitinternational.net/.

30. I am grateful to researcher Doug Wussler who discussed the topic of suicide in nuanced detail in the Good Death Society Blog (a project of Final Exit Network) on July 24, 2022.

31. Lonny Shavelson, *Medical Aid in Dying: A Guide for Patients and their Supporters*, published by the American Clinicians Academy on Medical Aid in Dying, 2022.

32. To learn more about the Exit Guide Program, contact them through their website: www.finalexitnetwork.org/connect-with-us.

33. https://finalexitnetwork.org/.

34. For more self-deliverance information, read Derek Humphry's *Final Exit: The Practicalities of Self-Deliverance and Assisted Suicide for the Dying*, https://finalexitnetwork.org/resources/final-exit-by-derek-humphry/.

35. Listserv discussion on May 3, 2022, on ACAMAID, www.acamaid.org.

Chapter 9

1. The Near Death Experience (NDE) literature is rife with reports from people who have died temporarily.

2. Dan Morhaim, *Preparing for a Better End: Expert Lessons on Death and Dying for You and Your Loved Ones* (Baltimore, MD: Johns Hopkins University Press, 2020), 132.

3. See www.bkbooks.com.

4. See also Chris Palmer, *Finding Meaning and Success: Living a Full and Productive Life* (Washington, DC: Rowman & Littlefield, 2021).

5. Barbara Karnes, *The Final Act of Living* (Vancouver, WA: Barbara Karnes Books, 2012), 27.

6. Christopher Kerr, medical director of Hospice of Buffalo, has written a lot about the visions and dreams that people, toward the end of life, may experience.

7. Barbara Karnes, *By Your Side: A Guide for Caring for the Dying at Home* (Vancouver, WA: Barbara Karnes Books, 2022).

8. Barbara Karnes, *By Your Side: A Guide for Caring for the Dying at Home* (Vancouver, WA: Barbara Karnes Books, 2022), 26.

9. I'm grateful to Sallie Tisdale whose 2018 book *Advice for Future Corpses* is illuminating. Her Chapter 4 discusses in detail how to talk with the very sick and inspired this

paragraph. See Sallie Tisdale, *Advice for Future Corpses: A Practical Perspective on Death and Dying* (New York: Touchstone, 2018).

10. See https://www.joincake.com/blog/winnie-the-pooh-quotes-about-loss/.

11. Michael Williams is a Before I Go Solutions senior end-of-life planning facilitator and trainer. He is also a storyteller and story coach and has a particular interest in legacy/life stories. See https://beforeigosolutions.com/michael-williams-3/.

12. See Barbara Karnes's blog for May 12, 2022, www.bkbooks.com.

13. Barbara Karnes, *By Your Side: A Guide for Caring for the Dying at Home* (Vancouver, WA: Barbara Karnes Books, 2022), 37.

14. See description of signs of active dying at https://www.vitas.com/for-healthcare -professionals/making-the-rounds/2020/march/signs-of-active-dying.

15. Katy Butler, *The Art of Dying Well: A Practical Guide to a Good End of Life* (New York: Scribner, 2019), 191.

CHAPTER 10

1. See www.greenburialcouncil.org.

2. Lancet Commission on the Value of Death, https://www.thelancet.com/commissions /value-of-death.

3. Drew Gilpin Faust, *The Republic of Suffering: Death and the American Civil War* (New York: Vintage Books, 2008), 92–96.

4. Drew Gilpin Faust, *The Republic of Suffering: Death and the American Civil War* (New York: Vintage Books, 2008), 93.

5. Jessica Mitford, *The American Way of Death Revisited* (New York: Vintage Books, 1998).

6. Jessica Mitford, *The American Way of Death Revisited* (New York: Vintage Books, 1998), 134–37.

7. Michael Hebb, *Let's Talk about Death over Dinner: An Invitation and Guide to Life's Most Important Conversation* (New York: Hachette Book Group, 2018), 56.

8. Quoted on page113 of Mark Shatz and Mel Helitzer, *Comedy Writing Secrets*, 3rd ed. (New York: Penguin Random House, 2016).

9. Caitlin Doughty, *Smoke Gets in Your Eyes: And Other Lessons from the Crematory* (New York: W. W. Norton & Company, 2014), 114 (italics in the original).

10. Caitlin Doughty, *Smoke Gets in Your Eyes: And Other Lessons from the Crematory* (New York: W. W. Norton & Company, 2014), 114.

11. The insightful quotes from Thomas Lynch come from Washington Post reporter Karen Heller in her essay on cremation in the *The Washington Post* on April 19, 2022.

12. See https://funerals.org/.

13. See https://mdfunerals.org/.

14. Full disclosure: I serve as vice president on FCAME's board.

15. Joshua Slocum and Lisa Carlson, *Final Rights: Reclaiming the American Way of Death* (Hinesburg, VT: Upper Access, Inc., Book Publishers, 2011).

16. Consumers can purchase grave packages that include all these items up front versus just the grave plot. Also, remember that purchasing a grave site means purchasing the rights to interment in that grave site rather than purchasing the land itself.

17. See https://mcusercontent.com/dde9c6af68c05540fcebc4835/files/eba12ff6-6c73 -be95-93c2-0ed494ad03b7/Funeral_Home_Online_Pricing_Report_6_21_22.pdf.

18. Jessica Mitford, *The American Way of Death Revisited* (New York: Vintage Books, 1998), 45.

19. Jessica Mitford, *The American Way of Death Revisited* (New York: Vintage Books, 1998), 43.

20. Caitlin Doughty, *Smoke Gets in Your Eyes: And Other Lessons from the Crematory* (New York: W. W. Norton & Company, 2014), 79.

21. See *New York Times*, https://www.nytimes.com/2011/07/21/business/despite -cancer-risk-embalmers-stay-with-formaldehyde.html.

22. Caitlin Doughty, *Smoke Gets in Your Eyes: And Other Lessons from the Crematory* (New York: W. W. Norton & Company, 2014), 80.

23. Caitlin Doughty, *Smoke Gets in Your Eyes: And Other Lessons from the Crematory* (New York: W. W. Norton & Company, 2014), 81.

24. Sallie Tisdale, *Advice for Future Corpses: A Practical Perspective on Death and Dying* (New York: Touchstone, 2018), 159.

25. Caitlin Doughty, *Smoke Gets in Your Eyes: And Other Lessons from the Crematory* (New York: W. W. Norton & Company, 2014), 116.

26. Caitlin Doughty, *Smoke Gets in Your Eyes: And Other Lessons from the Crematory* (New York: W. W. Norton & Company, 2014), 118, 119.

27. Barbara Blaylock, private email to the author, February 12, 2023.

28. I'm grateful to my friend Margaret Engel, the author and playwright, for this information. She sent it to me in a private email on July 8, 2023.

29. See https://www.angelenovalley.com/grave-liners-vs-burial-vaults.

30. See https://www.greenburialcouncil.org/.

31. See www.naturaldeath.org.uk.

32. Sallie Tisdale, *Advice for Future Corpses: A Practical Perspective on Death and Dying* (New York: Touchstone, 2018), 178.

33. See Caitlin Doughty, "If You Want to Give Something Back to Nature, Give Your Body," *New York Times*, December 5, 2022.

34. See Caitlin Doughty, "If You Want to Give Something Back to Nature, Give Your Body," *New York Times*, December 5, 2022.

35. Some of these names are trademarked.

36. The liquid byproduct of water cremation is a nontoxic solution of amino acids, peptides, sugars, and soap, which makes a wonderful fertilizer. Be a Tree Cremation in Denver, Colorado, calls this liquid Tree Tea™. Families may take some Tree Tea™ home to water trees and plants in their personal garden. Any remaining will be used on flowers and other nonedible plants. See https://www.beatreecremation.com/water-cremation.

37. Lauren Oster, "Could Water Cremation Become the New American Way of Death?," *Smithsonian Magazine*, July 27, 2022.

38. https://recompose.life/faqs/what-happens-to-drugs-and-medicine-during-human -composting/.

39. See Caitlin Doughty, "If You Want to Give Something Back to Nature, Give Your Body," *New York Times*, December 5, 2022.

40. See https://nfda.org/news/statistics.

41. For example, Sister Damien Marie Savino, a member of the Sisters of Saint Dominic of Amityville; Dr. Tobian Winright, Saint Louis University; Dr. Erin Lothes Biviano, College of St. Elizabeth in New Jersey; and Dr. Daniel Scheid at Duquesne University.

42. https://aboutplacejournal.org/issues/navigations-a-place-for-peace/gratitude/donelle-dreese/.

43. For more information about conservation burial, see the Conservation Burial Alliance website www.conservationburialalliance.org.

44. The phrase "back to the future" comes from the title of a popular science-fiction film released in 1985. The movie, directed by Robert Zemeckis and produced by Steven Spielberg, is called *Back to the Future*. It stars Michael J. Fox as Marty McFly and Christopher Lloyd as Dr. Emmett "Doc" Brown. The film's plot revolves around time travel, where Marty McFly accidentally travels back in time from 1985 to 1955 using a time-traveling DeLorean car invented by Dr. Brown. Throughout the movie, Marty must navigate the challenges of being in the past and find a way to return to the future. The phrase "back to the future" encapsulates the central theme of the film, which is the idea of traveling backward in time and then back to one's original timeline. The film was a massive success and became a pop-culture icon, spawning two sequels, *Back to the Future Part II* (1989) and *Back to the Future Part III* (1990). The trilogy has remained popular over the years, and the phrase "back to the future" has become synonymous with the concept of time travel and revisiting the past or bringing aspects from the past into the present or future contexts.

45. See https://www.homefuneralalliance.org/.

46. See http://homefuneralalliance.org/.

47. https://inelda.org/.

48. https://www.nedalliance.org/.

49. See this free video from Lee Webster: https://vimeo.com/638792393?share=copy.

50. See https://www.homefuneralalliance.org/.

51. Joshua Slocum and Lisa Carlson, *Final Rights: Reclaiming the American Way of Death* (Hinesburg, VT: Upper Access, Inc., Book Publishers, 2011), 129.

52. See earlier in the book on page 83 for more discussion of organ donation.

CHAPTER 11

1. Many articles and books give good advice on how to plan a memorial service. One of the best is from the Funeral Consumers Alliance. See *How to Plan a Memorial Service* at https://funerals.org/?consumers=planning-memorial-service.

2. There are many books and articles on how to write a eulogy. One of the best articles is from Jennifer Calonia with Grammarly in an article entitled *How to Write a Eulogy*, March 24, 2022, https://www.grammarly.com/blog/how-to-write-a-eulogy/.

3. Jill Werman Harris, *Remembrances and Celebrations: A Book of Eulogies, Elegies, Letters, and Epitaphs* (New York: Pantheon Books, 1999), xvii.

4. I'm grateful to many sources on obituaries. One of the best is an essay by Angela Morrow, RN, entitled *How to Write an Obituary*, October 11, 2022, https://www.verywellhealth.com/how-to-write-an-obituary-1132597#toc-how-to-write-an-obituary-step-by-step.

5. I'm grateful to journalist and author Margaret Engel for this information, which she sent me in a private email on July 8, 2023.

CHAPTER 12

1. Barbara Coombs Lee, *Finish Strong: Putting Your Priorities First at Life's End* (Portland, OR: Compassion & Choices, 2019), 56.

2. https://bkbooks.com/blogs/something-to-think-about/stuck-in-grief.

3. Joan Didion, *The Year of Magical Thinking* (New York: Alfred A. Knopf, 2005), 27.

4. Joan Didion, *The Year of Magical Thinking* (New York: Alfred A. Knopf, 2005), 188.

5. This information about normal grief reactions comes from my work as a hospice volunteer and from Montgomery Hospice and Prince George's Hospice in Montgomery County, Maryland. Disclosure: I serve on its board.

6. Full disclosure: I serve on the board of the Montgomery Hospice and Prince George's Hospice in Maryland, United States.

7. A useful resource here is Brene Brown, *Atlas of the Heart: Mapping Meaningful Connection and the Language of Human Experience* (New York: Random House, 2021), 110–13.

8. Jill Bialosky, "Grief Is a Forever Thing," *New York Times*, December 4, 2022.

9. See https://www.britannica.com/summary/Harriet-Beecher-Stowe.

10. Sarah Murray, *Making an Exit: From the Magnificent to the Macabre—How We Dignify the Dead* (New York: St. Martin's Press, 2011), 155.

11. David Kessler, *Finding Meaning: The Sixth Stage of Grief* (New York: Scribner, 2019), 2.

12. BJ Miller and Shoshana Berger, *A Beginner's Guide to the End: Practical Advice for Living Life and Facing Death* (New York: Simon & Schuster, 2019), 135.

13. An excellent guide on grief is the following special report from the Harvard Medical School, *Grief and Loss: A Guide to Preparing for and Mourning the Death of a Loved One*, published in 2017.

14. Jane Brody, "Making Meaning Out of Grief," *New York Times*, November 5, 2019.

15. Ann Bennet, private email to the author, June 6, 2023.

16. See https://www.theatlantic.com/health/archive/2014/03/in-grief-try-personal-rituals/284397/.

EPILOGUE

1. Chris Matthews, *American: Beyond Our Grandest Notions* (New York: Free Press, 2002).

2. https://poemanalysis.com/emily-dickinson/that-it-will-never-come-again/.

3. Irvin Yalom, *Becoming Myself: A Psychiatrist's Memoir* (New York: Basic Books, 2017), 288.

4. Irvin Yalom, *Staring at the Sun: Overcoming the Dread of Death* (Boston: Little Brown, 2008), 147.

5. Meredith Taylor, private email to the author, December 22, 2022.

6. For more on developing a vision for one's life, see my book *Finding Meaning and Success: Living a Fulfilled and Productive Life* (Washington, DC: Rowman & Littlefield, 2021).

7. I highly recommend Dr. Mardy Grothe and his many books. His website is www .drmardy.com, and his free weekly e-newsletter is a gem.

8. For more on the meaning of life, see Chris Palmer, *Finding Meaning and Success: Living a Fulfilled and Productive Life* (Washington, DC: Rowman & Littlefield, 2021).

9. Katharine Esty, *Eightysomethings: A Practical Guide to Letting Go, Aging Well, and Finding Unexpected Happiness* (Brattleboro, VT: Skyhorse Publishing, 2019), 164.

10. Irvin Yalom, *Becoming Myself: A Psychiatrist's Memoir* (New York: Basic Books, 2017), 294.

11. Lev Tolstoy, *The Death of Ivan Ilych* (Jerusalem, Israel: Minerva Publishing, 2018, first published in 1886).

12. Dr. Atul Gawande, *Being Mortal: Medicine and What Matters in the End* (New York: Henry Holt and Company, Metropolitan Books, 2014), 2.

13. BJ Miller and Shoshana Berger, *A Beginner's Guide to the End: Practical Advice for Living Life and Facing Death* (New York: Simon & Schuster, 2019).

14. Michael Hebb, *Let's Talk about Death (over Dinner): An Invitation and Guide to Life's Most Important Conversation* (New York: Hachette Book Group, 2018), 94.

15. Sheldon Solomon, Jeff Greenberg, and Tom Pyszczynski, *On the Role of Death in Life: The Worm at the Core* (New York: Random House, 2015), 225.

16. Irvin Yalom, *Becoming Myself: A Psychiatrist's Memoir* (New York: Basic Books, 2017), 338.

17. Irvin Yalom, *Staring at the Sun: Overcoming the Dread of Death* (Boston: Little Brown, 2008), 35.

18. Full disclosure: I worked in the Carter administration.

19. Hank Dunn, *Hard Choices for Loving People: CPR, Feeding Tubes, Palliative Care, Comfort Measures, and the Patient with a Serious Illness*, www.hankdunn.com, 2016, 53.

20. Katy Butler, *The Art of Dying Well: A Practical Guide to a Good End of Life* (New York: Scribner, 2019).

21. Hank Dunn, *Hard Choices for Loving People: CPR, Feeding Tubes, Palliative Care, Comfort Measures, and the Patient with a Serious Illness*, www.hankdunn.com, 2016, 4.

22. Haider Warraich, *Modern Death: How Medicine Changed the End of Life* (New York: St. Martin's Press, 2017), 264.

23. Daniel Callahan, *The Troubled Dream of Life: In Search of a Peaceful Death* (Washington, DC: Georgetown University Press, 2000), 229.

24. Jessica Nutik Zitter, *Extreme Measures: Finding a Better Path to the End of Life* (New York: Penguin Random House, 2017), 48.

25. Dr. Louise Aronson, *Elderhood: Redefining Aging, Transforming Medicine, Reimagining Life* (London: Bloomsbury Publishing, 2019), 148.

26. Derek Humphry, *Final Exit: The Practicalities of Self-Deliverance and Assisted Suicide for the Dying* (McHenry, IL: Delta Trade Paperback, 2010), xiv.

27. Chris Palmer and Christina Palmer, MD, *Open Heart: When Open-Heart Surgery Becomes Your Best Option* (Rockville, MD: Bethesda Communications Group, 2021).

28. Isaac Asimov, *Asimov Laughs Again: More Than 700 Favorite Jokes, Limericks, and Anecdotes* (New York: Harper Collins Publishers, 1972), 341.

29. I'm grateful to author and psychiatrist Irvin Yalom for the notion of an awakening. For example, see Yalom's book *Staring at the Sun: Overcoming the Dread of Death* (Boston: Little Brown, 2008), 35.

INDEX

alkaline hydrolysis (water crema-
tion), 166–67
allow natural death (AND), 24,
82, 223
Alzheimer's, 18, 71, 123–24,
133, 136
Ameche, Brian, 132–33
American (Matthews), 197
American Academy of Family
Physicians, 131
American Academy of Hospice
and Palliative Medicine, 131
American Cancer Society
(ACS), 38
American Clinicians Academy
on Medical Aid in Dying
(ACAMAID), 128
American College of Legal
Medicine, 131
American Nurses Association, 131
American Public Health
Association, 131
Americans with Disabilities
Act, 135
The American Way of Death
(Mitford), 154–55, 158
AND (allow natural death), 24,
82, 223
Angelou, Maya, 248
anticipatory grief, 98, 191
Applewhite, Ashton, 44
aquamation (water cremation),
166–67
Aronson, Louise, 43, 80, 208
arrival, of death, 148

Ars Moriendi (the "art of dying"),
35, 198
The Art of Dying Well (Butler, K.),
36, 206, 214
Asimov, Isaac, 5, 211
Asimov Laughs Again
(Asimov), 211
"assisted suicide," 133, 134, 138
The Atlantic (magazine), 198
At Peace (Harrington), 22, 83
attorney, power of, 56, 57, 58,
59, 74
audience, legacy letters, 89–90
Australia, euthanasia in, 133–34
autobiographies, 92–93
"awakening experience," life as,
199, 212
Aziz, Shahid, 68, 77, 126

Baby Boom generation, 77, 104
"back to the future," burials, 172
bad (hard) deaths: COVID-
19 and, 8–9; examples, 11, 14,
15, 17–18, 66, 78, 201–2, 205;
in ICUs, 9, 16–17, 25–26, 68,
205, 223. *See also* good deaths
bathing ceremony, honoring and,
3, 148–49, 178, 224–25
Beacon Hill Village, Boston, 46
beautiful death, 141, 204
The Beauty of Dusk (Bruni), 33
Becker, Joshua, 55–56
before death (living) funeral,
178, 256

129–30, 131, 132, 136; VSED and, 121, 123, 132, 214, 223

Medical Aid in Dying (Shavelson), 135

Medical Evaluation Committee, FEN, 137

medical organizations, with MAID, 131

medical/physician order for life-sustaining treatment (MOLST/POLST), 23, 81–82, 223–24

medical providers, 6, 137, 143; with death made official, 148–49; ICUs and moral distress of, 26; palliative care team, 106, 108–9, 112, 122; wrongful-prolongation-of-life lawsuits, 73–74, 218, 224. *See also* caregivers; doctors; nurses, hospice

medical treatments: aggressive, 83, 109; "conveyor belt" of, 9, 30, 109, 208; dementia and line to withhold, 71, 121; financial incentives with, 20–21; MOLST/POLST, 23, 81–82, 223–24; with negligible benefits, 108, 198; overtreating, 18–21, 38, 79, 108, 216–18; surgeries, 9, 20–23, 108, 206; technology, 4, 20, 28–29, 71, 120, 127, 205–6, 213, 217; unwanted life-sustaining,

120–21, 218. *See also* cardiopulmonary resuscitation

Medicare, 60, 62–63, 77, 79, 107–8, 115

medication, ingesting MAID, 135–36

medicine: "defensive," 20; donation of bodies for, 175; fast, 30–31; slow, 29–32

memento mori (remembering we will die), 5–6, 37

memoirs, 42, 85, 92–95

memorial services: eulogists, 257; funeral service versus, 178–79; invitees and guests, 256; memory table with significant "physical things," 260; music, 61, 257, 258–60; notes for, 61, 256–60; officiant or funeral celebrant, 257; organizing, 179; photos, 260; postcards for written stories, 257; programs, 179, 257–58; purpose and role of, 179; readings, 258, 261–62; venue, 256

memory: care facility, 75; of how people die, 143; legacy letters, 232–35, 240–41; memoirs, 42, 85, 92–95; remembering, 5–6, 37, 94–95, 190, 199, 203, 258, 261; table at memorial services, 260. *See also* dementia

mental life goals, 42

Menzel, Paul, 121–22, 124, 138

microbial decomposition, 167

About the Author

Chris Palmer is an author, speaker, wildlife filmmaker, conservationist, professor, and grandfather. He dedicated his professional career to conservation but now devotes his life to death and dying issues. He is a trained hospice volunteer and founded and runs an aging, death, and dying group for the Bethesda Metro Area Village where he is also a board member. He frequently gives presentations and workshops on aging, death, and dying issues—he is an end-of-life activist.

He serves as vice chairperson of the board of Montgomery Hospice & Prince George's Hospice, is vice president of the board of the Funeral Consumers Alliance of Maryland & Environs, and serves on the Advisory Council for the Maryland Office of Cemetery Oversight. He also serves on the boards of Final Exit Network, Funeral Consumers Alliance, and Hemlock Society of San Diego. He was formerly a board member of the Green Burial Association of Maryland.

Chris and his wife, Gail Shearer, have created and funded the "Finishing Strong Award" with the Washington Area Village Exchange (WAVE) to encourage villages to hold more discussions about end-of-life issues. WAVE is the largest regional village organization in the nation.

Chris also serves as president of the MacGillivray Freeman Films Educational Foundation, producing and funding IMAX films on science and conservation issues. MacGillivray Freeman Films is the world's largest and most successful producer of IMAX films.

During his filmmaking career, he swam with dolphins and whales, came face-to-face with sharks and Kodiak bears, camped with wolf packs, and waded hip-deep through Everglade swamps. For over thirty-five years, he spearheaded the production of more than three hundred hours of original programming for prime-time television and the IMAX film industry, winning him and his colleagues many awards, including two Emmys and an Oscar nomination. He has worked with Robert Redford, Paul Newman, Jane Fonda, Ted Turner, and many other celebrities. His IMAX films include *Whales, Wolves, Dolphins, Bears, Coral Reef Adventure*, and *Grand Canyon Adventure*.

He has written ten books, including *Finding Meaning and Success: Living a Fulfilled and Productive Life*, published by Rowman & Littlefield in 2021—all proceeds from Chris's books fund scholarships for American University students. Starting in 2004, Chris served on American University's full-time faculty as Distinguished Film Producer in Residence until his retirement in 2018. While at American University, he founded and directed the Center for Environmental Filmmaking at the School of Communication. He also created and taught a popular class called Design Your Life for Success.

Chris and Gail have lived in Bethesda, Maryland, for nearly fifty years and raised three daughters. They now have nine grandchildren. Chris was a stand-up comic for five years and has advanced degrees from University College London and Harvard. He has jumped out of helicopters, worked on an Israeli kibbutz, and was a high-school boxing champion. Chris is currently learning to juggle, draw, dance, play tennis, and play the piano. He loves standing on his hands for exercise and keeps a daily gratitude journal. His website is www.ChrisPalmerOnline.com, and his email is christopher.n.palmer@gmail.com.